HOW TO COPE
SUCCESSFULLY WITH

HIGH BLOOD PRESSURE

DR DUNCAN DYMOND

Wellhouse Publishing Ltd

First published in Great Britain in 2003 by
Wellhouse Publishing Ltd
31 Middle Bourne Lane
Lower Bourne
Farnham
Surrey GU10 3NH

© Duncan Dymond 2003

Duncan Dymond asserts the moral right to be
identified as the author of this work.

DISCLAIMER

The aim of this book is to provide general information only and
should not be treated as a substitute for the medical advice of
your doctor or any other health care professional. The publisher
and author is not responsible or liable for any diagnosis made by
a reader based on the contents of this book. Always consult your
doctor if you are in any way concerned about your health.

A catalogue record for this book is available from the British Library

ISBN 1 903784 07 7

Printed and bound in Great Britain by
Biddles Ltd., Surrey. www.biddles.co.uk

Contents

Foreword

High blood pressure is just about the most common medical condition in the developed world, and as access to medical care improves in the developing countries more and more people are being discovered to suffer from it world-wide.

Patients with high blood pressure fill GPs' surgeries, cardiology clinics, and the clinics of kidney specialists, vascular specialists, eye specialists and neurologists. It is a silent killer, responsible for wrecking millions of lives. In this book I have tried to explain in simple language the importance and mechanisms of high blood pressure, and how high blood pressure is defined, investigated and treated. I have also tried to lay to rest some of the myths that continue to do the rounds.

Duncan Dymond

Chapter One

Introduction

'I've got blood pressure, doctor' is a common opening remark in the dialogue between patient and doctor. 'Blood Pressure' is not a heart disease. In fact it is not a disease at all, and we should be thankful that we have a blood pressure, for without it we could not be alive.

When we talk about blood pressure we are referring to the pressure that keeps the blood circulating through our arteries to deliver blood to all our organs. If we slithered around like snakes, walked around on all fours like cats or if our brains were more or less on the same level as our hearts, then a low pressure would be needed to deliver the blood from the heart to the brain. Imagine what would happen if we suddenly stood upright: this low level of pressure would be insufficient to send the blood up to our heads and we would lose consciousness and fall over. With our heads so far above our hearts we need a higher level of pressure than a cat or a dog to send blood to the brain - giraffes require a pressure that is higher still!

Blood pressure, or the pressure in the arteries, can be compared to the pressure required in a central heating system to send hot water from the boiler to the radiators in the upper floors of a house. Your heart is akin to the pump of the central heating system, the driving force that delivers blood around the body. The height of the blood pressure will depend both on the amount of blood that is pumped out by the heart with each beat, and also how vigorous or strong the heart muscle is.

However, the heart is far from being the ruling force in the control of blood pressure. As doctors have learned more about the causes of high blood pressure, it is now known that the heart is not nearly as important as the arterial system (sometimes known as the arterial tree) in the body.

Let us imagine that the heart pumps 5 litres per minute around the body. If the arteries in the body are nicely relaxed and dilated (expanded), then the pressure in those arteries will be low, but if the arteries become narrowed or constricted, then the same 5 litres a minute will produce a much higher resistance, and hence a higher pressure.

The concept of resistance to flow being related to the diameter of the blood vessels can easily be illustrated using the example of a garden hose. If you turn the hose full on and just let the water flow out through the end of the hose, then the stream may run for about a foot before falling to the ground. Now attach an adjustable nozzle that enables you to project the water for several feet in front of you onto distant flowerbeds. By adjusting the nozzle to achieve the maximum distance, you are in fact narrowing the orifice through which the water will flow so that it comes out at much higher pressure and will travel further.

The open garden hose, therefore, represents your arteries when they are dilated or relaxed; the nozzle, at its tightest, represents the arteries when they are constricted. The tight hose nozzle is a high-resistance system that produces high pressure, and the open hose is a low-resistance system which equates to low pressure. In the body, it is the resistance produced by the arteries which dictates the blood pressure. Abnormally high resistance will make the blood pressure too high, causing high blood pressure (also known as hypertension).

The Arterioles

It is not the largest arteries in the body which control resistance, but the smaller ones known as arterioles. These arterioles are controlled by many complex systems within the body, and it is quite normal for resistance in the arterioles to vary from organ to organ depending upon what we are doing. For example, after a meal the digestive system needs more blood, whereas the muscles need less. Resistance in the arterioles that deliver blood to the intestines will therefore be reduced, enabling blood flow to be diverted there, whilst arterioles in the muscles will constrict so blood is sent away from the muscles to where it is most needed. When we exercise, our hearts beat faster to increase the amount of blood travelling around the arterial system, but the arterioles supplying the muscles in the legs and arms will dilate, reducing resistance there, while blood flow to the intestines will be lowered.

This regulatory mechanism of the arterioles helps us survive major

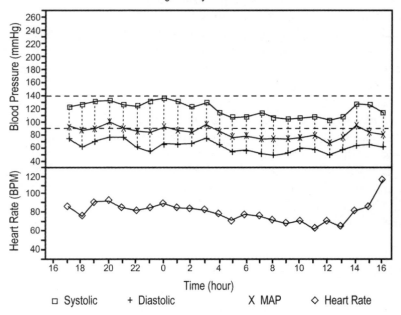

Figure 1.1

A 24-hour blood pressure print-out from a patient with normal blood pressure. The dotted lines represent normal systolic and diastolic pressures of 140mm and 90mm of mercury (Hg) respectively. The small squares are the systolic pressures, and the crosses diastolic pressures. The 'x's are average pressures (MAP), and the diamonds are the heart rates over the monitoring period. Note that all the systolic and diastolic readings are below their respective dotted lines, and note also how both readings fall at night during sleep.

trauma such as blood loss. If we have an accident and lose a substantial amount of blood, then blood flow must be preserved for the essential organs - namely the brain, the heart and the kidneys - to keep us alive. Arterioles to the skin and muscles will constrict so that what blood is left can be pumped at sufficient pressure to keep the brain, the heart and the kidneys working. This explains why someone who has lost a lot of blood has such cold skin.

In patients who have abnormally high blood pressure, a persistently raised resistance in the arterioles is the major abnormality. The causes of this will be explained in Chapter Three

Blood pressure is therefore not constant, and will change continuously depending upon the amount of blood pumped out by the heart and the resistance in the blood vessels. Blood pressure will fall while we are asleep and horizontal, and go up when we are active and upright. Figure 1.1 shows a print-out from a 24-hour blood pressure monitor showing the top and bottom readings and how they change when we are awake and when we are asleep (I will return to the definitions of the top and bottom readings below).

In patients with high blood pressure, the surges in pressure that occur on waking and in the morning hours may be responsible for the higher incidence of heart attacks and strokes at these times of the day (see Chapter Five).

Upper and Lower Readings

Even if you have never had your blood pressure measured, you probably know that doctors refer to blood pressure as two numbers. The upper reading is known as 'systolic' and the lower reading as 'diastolic'. Both numbers are expressed in millimetres of mercury (mm/Hg). So in a blood pressure reading of 120/80, 120 is the systolic pressure, 80 the diastolic. The systolic reading is the peak pressure generated in the arterial tree by each heartbeat. The diastolic reading is the lowest to which the pressure falls when the heart is relaxing between beats. The two words are derived from Greek, meaning 'contraction' and 'relaxation' respectively. When your doctor refers to a pressure of '120 over 80', this means the systolic reading is 120 millimetres of mercury and the diastolic is 80 millimetres of mercury.

It is very common for patients to have heard through a medical grapevine that 'the lower reading is more important than the higher one'.

I do not know how the myth became established in medical folklore that the diastolic reading is more important than the systolic, but there is certainly no good medical explanation for it. Researchers have known for at least 40 years that both the systolic and diastolic pressures are important for predicting the future risk of heart attacks, strokes or some other vascular disaster. In fact, once you get to your mid-forties, the systolic pressure is probably more important than the diastolic in predicting such risk.

Systolic pressure tends to rise with advancing age, particularly in the Western world. Many people regard this as normal, although some blood pressure experts disagree. It is interesting that systolic pressure does not rise to such a degree in elderly people from developing countries, although the reasons for this are not clear (this piece of medical spin means 'doctors don't have a clue'). However, doctors are now increasingly aware of the importance of treating high systolic pressures in the older patient, as this is beneficial in preventing heart attacks and strokes. I will return to this in Chapter Nine.

Now that we have established that having a measurable blood pressure means you are alive and kicking, let us move on to high blood pressure and what it means.

Chapter Two

High Blood Pressure – What Is It?

High blood pressure is known as hypertension (hyper = too much, tension = pressure). It is generally believed that about 2,000 years ago a wise Chinese emperor noticed that people who had very strong pulses suffered from strokes. This incredibly observant emperor also noticed that people who ate a lot of salt had strong and bounding pulses. It seems appropriate to regard this emperor as the first person to recognise the complications of high blood pressure.

Measuring Blood Pressure

Around 1730, a biologist and curate named Steven Hales made the first direct measurement of blood pressure. He put a catheter into an artery of a horse and measured the height of the column of blood rising up a tube of glass. He noticed that when the horse was under stress (such as that caused by having a tube put into an artery!), its blood pressure went up. This direct measurement of blood pressure - placing a tube into arteries - has also been used for research in humans, although fortunately we now have less invasive ways of measuring it.

In 1827 an eminent physician called Dr Bright noticed that people with end-stage kidney failure had large hearts; he inferred that they must have high blood pressure, although of course at that time he could not actually make any measurements.

The first indirect measurement of blood pressure that did not involve sticking a needle into an artery became possible thanks to an invention by Scipione Rocci. Using a mercury-based manometer (pressure-measuring system), he measured the pressure needed to obliterate the pulse at the wrist when a cuff was pumped up around the arm. The principle of pumping up a cuff and measuring the pressure where the pulse disappears is still used today. We owe the discovery of actually listening to the artery rather than feeling it to a Russian

Army surgeon called Korotkov. He noted that various sounds could be heard as the mercury manometer was deflated. The mercury-based blood pressure machine has stood the test of time, although digital and electronic devices have meant that they are gradually being phased out. One reason mercury machines are being replaced is that they are regarded as environmentally unfriendly.

As explained in Chapter One, the blood pressure is expressed as two readings, and these may be measured from the appearance and disappearance of the sound of the pulse using a blood pressure machine (the standard mercury-based one is known as a *sphygmo-manometer* - often abbreviated to 'asphyxia'). The doctor will pump the cuff up around the patient's upper arm. The correct way is to pump the cuff up gently with a finger over the pulse in the elbow or wrist, and only to pump it to about 10-20mm of mercury above where the pulse is no longer felt.

With the stethoscope placed over the artery in the crease of the elbow, the cuff should be deflated very slowly and a note will be made of when the sound of the pulse returns. This is recorded as the systolic pressure. When the sound of the pulse disappears, this is noted down as the diastolic pressure reading.

Blood pressure may be measured with the patient sitting or lying down, but rarely with the patient standing up. Sometimes a patient may have come to see the doctor because he or she suffers dizziness when standing up; in these cases doctors will usually measure the pressure with the patient lying down *and* standing, to see if the pressure falls when the patient is upright.

The body normally uses complex regulatory mechanisms to make sure that blood pressure does not fall when we stand up. The reason for this is that blood flow to the brain has to be preserved to at all costs, otherwise when we stand up the blood flow to our brains would drop and we would faint. The condition of feeling dizzy or having a blood pressure drop when we change from being seated or lying down to standing up is known as 'postural hypotension'. This is very common in the elderly, whose regulatory mechanisms may not be as good as those in younger patients, and it may also be seen in some rare neurological conditions, and also occasionally in people with diabetes. In the old days, when only a few drugs were available to treat high blood pressure, postural hypotension was a common side-effect, which understandably made these drugs immensely unpopular with patients.

As a general rule it does not matter in which arm blood pressure is measured, as it should be more or less the same on both sides.

Blood pressure is a dynamic measurement dependent both on the pumping action of the heart and how dilated or constricted the arteries are. It would therefore be highly unlikely for blood pressure to remain the same from minute to minute or from hour to hour. So, if you go into your doctor to have your blood pressure checked having just rushed in from work, been buffeted on the tube or bus, or sat stranded in a traffic jam for hours, then you should not be surprised if your blood pressure is high! Similarly, if you have your blood pressure measured after lying down in a darkened room for an hour listening to relaxing music, then you should not be surprised if it is lower than normal. Our blood pressure reflects our general state of mental and physical agitation. Doctors should recognise this when trying to interpret any one reading at any particular time.

You may have had your blood pressure measured and be familiar with the 'sphygmo' - a wooden or metal box containing the mercury column and the cuff and tubing that go with it. You would think that such a simple system would be relatively error-free, but this is not the case. If the rubber tubing is perished and leaky, the readings may be artificially low. One of the most common causes of mistakes apart from old equipment, a faulty stethoscope (or a deaf doctor!) is the actual size of the cuff. If the cuff is too small, then the blood pressure may read too high. The tendency for doctors now to be given Velcro cuffs rather than cuffs that tuck in can exacerbate this problem. Cuffs for large arms are available, therefore if you feel the cuff giving way or if your doctor is struggling to keep a grip on the cuff on your arm, then you might politely ask him or her if a larger cuff might not be more appropriate.

The Heart and High Blood Pressure

Although many patients with high blood pressure may be referred to a cardiologist, let me reiterate that having high blood pressure does not mean that you are a cardiac patient or that you have heart disease. It is the state of the arteries and whether they are over-constricted or relaxed that dictates the blood pressure. This state of

...al constriction or relaxation is known as 'tone', and is under the influence of several different mechanisms in the body.

The heart should be regarded as one of the innocent victims of high blood pressure. It is the *consequences* of high blood pressure that damage the heart and other organs such as the kidneys and the brain, and also the aorta. If the heart were the main culprit in producing high blood pressure, then we might expect the magnificent heart muscle of a highly trained athlete to produce higher blood pressure than that of a patient who has suffered one or two heart attacks. In fact the athlete and the heart attack victim may have identical blood pressures. The reason is that, as mentioned in Chapter One, it is the *resistance to blood flow in the arterioles* that largely controls blood pressure.

The kidneys, rather than the heart, are much more blameworthy in most patients with high blood pressure. In the 1890s a scientist called Tigerstedt demonstrated the role of the kidneys in elevating blood pressure. In experiments that would no longer be regarded as acceptable, he mashed up some rabbit kidneys and injected the extract into four other rabbits. The blood pressure of the injected rabbits went up. We now know that a chemical called *renin* is manufactured deep within the cells of the kidneys. When renin gets into the blood plasma, it converts a chemical with the tongue-twisting name of angiotensinogen into another chemical called angiotensin I. Angiotensin I is immediately changed to angiotensin II by an enzyme called the angiotensin converting enzyme (ACE). (Some of you may be taking drugs known as ACE-inhibitors which stop the conversion of these chemicals - see Chapter Seven.)

Angiotensin II is an incredibly powerful constrictor of arteries, with many complex actions. Not only does it act directly on arteries, it also stimulates the adrenal glands (which are small glands that sit on top of each kidney) to produce another chemical called aldosterone. Aldosterone sends a signal to the kidneys to retain salt - so you can see that by producing renin, the kidneys induce actions involving constriction of the arteries and those involving salt-retention, and have a lot to answer for regarding high blood pressure.

Why does our body bother to manufacture renin? This is another in-built protective mechanism. If we are injured and lose a lot of blood, or if our blood pressure drops for any reason, then blood flow into the kidneys falls. This acts as a powerful stimulus for the kidneys to manufacture renin, to help us to retain salt and water and to constrict our arteries to keep the blood pressure up and blood flow to the essential organs preserved. It is possible that in some patients an overactivity of the renin and angiotensin system contributes to the development of high blood pressure, although it is very hard to prove this.

I will come back to the kidneys as the potential culprits of high blood pressure in Chapter Three.

How Do We Define Hypertension?

This is the cause of much debate, and even more confusion! There is still no universally-recognised definition of hypertension. There has been a concerted effort to find one because, as more is known about hypertension, and as better drugs with fewer side-effects have become available, more people are having their blood pressure measured more frequently, so we should at least have a definition. This is easier said than done, however. Definitions also have to take into account the fact that our population is ageing, so what is normal and desirable for a 30 year old may not necessarily be so for an octogenarian.

The World Health Organization and the British Hypertension Society have slightly different definitions of hypertension, but each in its own way tries to be pragmatic. The World Health Organization criteria regard a normal blood pressure as a systolic reading of less than 140mm of mercury and a diastolic reading less than 90mm of mercury. Borderline hypertension is a systolic of 140-159mm of mercury and/or diastolic readings of 90-94mm of mercury. Definite hypertension is defined as a systolic reading of 160mm of mercury or more and/or a diastolic reading of 95mm of mercury or more, with the adjective 'mild' hypertension describing readings of 160-179 systolic and/or diastolic readings of 95-104mm of mercury. These criteria are rather fixed and rigid, and do not take the patient's age into account, but some experts have suggested that in patients over 80 years of age hypertension might be defined as a diastolic pressure persistently greater than 100mm of mercury.

The point of the debate is not just so doctors can argue about numbers, but to come up with some sort of working definition for what, in the words of the late Professor Geoffrey Rose, is 'that level of blood pressure above which investigations and treatment do more good than harm'. Built into this sensible definition is the realisation that a certain level of blood pressure in one person with no other risk factors for heart disease and strokes, etc., may be far too high for another person with a whole host of additional risk factors. Doctors are therefore encouraged to look at the blood pressure reading as part of a holistic approach to a patient's overall vascular risk.

There are various computer programmes in a continuous state of evolution which allow doctors to key in a patient's risk factors and come up with a numerical value to predict the 10-year likelihood of the patient to have a heart attack or stroke. There are also charts, for people who are suspicious of computers. More information on this is given in Chapter Seven.

Some of the definitions of hypertension which have focused only on the diastolic pressure are obviously incomplete, because they do not take into account the systolic pressure. I mentioned in Chapter One the myth that diastolic pressure is much more important than systolic, whereas we now know that this is just not the case. Isolated systolic hypertension is a common condition in older people. As we get older our arteries become less elastic and they may become thicker. Systolic pressure may therefore be high even when the diastolic pressure is absolutely normal. Individuals with this condition have a higher risk of cardiovascular complications compared to younger hypertensive individuals, and we now believe that isolated systolic hypertension, as this situation is known, should be treated.

I will return to the British Hypertension Society guidelines for treating hypertension and the treatment of hypertension in the elderly in Chapter Nine.

What Are the Causes of Hypertension?

A simple question, you might think, but unfortunately there is no simple answer. We are probably no nearer to knowing exactly what makes any one individual suffer with high blood pressure than we are to knowing the origins of the universe. There are many theories.

Epidemiologists are doctors who study the incidence of disease in populations and who look at the frequency of diseases such as heart attacks and strokes in different groups depending upon their lifestyle and where they live. Epidemiological research first discovered the link between smoking and lung cancer. Epidemiologists have looked at the environmental factors that influence blood pressure and matched them up with genetic factors. They have also studied what happens to blood pressure when populations migrate from one part of the world to another.

Many people accept that their blood pressure will go up as a consequence of living to an advanced age, and it is certainly true that in Western countries older people have higher pressures than young people. This does not necessarily mean it is a 'normal' phenomenon. There appears to be a difference between the way blood pressure in the elderly rises in developed countries compared to those in developing countries. In some rural areas, particularly in Africa, high blood pressure is almost unheard of in elderly people. An interesting study from Kenya showed that when tribesmen with normal blood pressures in their rural communities migrate to Nairobi, their blood pressures rise! This would suggest that environmental factors might contribute to the development of high blood pressure as we get older. However, it may also give some logic to the advice doctors give their stressed-out patients with high blood pressure - to go and relax away from the pressures of work!

There is also some evidence that if we start with a higher blood pressure than normal in early life, our blood pressure will rise more quickly than that of our peers as we get older, although the causes of this are unclear.

Genetics and Family History

Most people with high blood pressure will know, or find out eventually, that one of their parents, grandparents, a brother or sister also has it, as it does tend to run in families. It is very convenient to blame a condition that we do not entirely understand on our parents. What we do not know is whether it is the genetic factors themselves that cause the hypertension, or whether there is some genetic predisposition to developing high blood pressure in any given environment. It has been suggested that someone who has a normal blood pressure but who has hypertension in the family may develop high blood pressure in response to stress, excess alcohol or excess salt. Someone else with a different family background can drink as much beer and eat as many crisps as he or she likes without developing high blood pressure.

A large study of over 400,000 Americans found there was a greater than one in three chance of developing hypertension if there was a family history of hypertension, but less than one in five chance if there was no family history. This is quite a big difference.

There are also racial differences in the incidence of high blood pressure. Hypertension is more common in people of African and Caribbean origin than in whites. As mentioned above, Africans living outside the cities have a lower blood pressure than their urban counterparts, but even in the developed world the incidence of hypertension in Africans and Caribbeans is higher than can be explained solely by changes in diet and economic conditions. Even the drugs we use to control high blood pressure in people of African and Caribbean origin are different from those used for other racial groups (see Chapter Eight).

Another ethnic group which has caught the imagination with regard to hypertension is the Japanese. In Japan, hypertension is extremely common, as are strokes. It has been suggested that there is something in the Japanese diet that predisposes them to high blood pressure. Interestingly enough, examination of Japanese populations moving to cities such as Los Angeles has shown that, as they adopt an American diet, their blood pressures go down but the incidence of heart attacks goes up! Perhaps the stress of the traffic jams and the smog in Los Angeles is more detrimental to health than the Japanese diet.

As mentioned above, the relationship of salt intake to blood pressure was noticed many years ago, and there are certainly modern studies that have shown that populations who consume little salt have hardly any hypertension. Conversely, groups with a high salt intake have higher blood pressures. As with any statistic, we have to be careful not to jump to conclusions. Until recently it would have been premature to say that a high salt intake was the definitive cause of hypertension. However, the Inter Salt Project, which looked at populations from 32 countries, did seem to show that the rise in blood pressure with advancing age was related to dietary salt. Therefore, the medical advice that people with high blood pressure should reduce the amount of salt in their diet now seems more like logic and less like mere whim.

What of Alcohol?

Many studies have shown that a high alcohol intake is associated with a high risk of having a stroke. There is no doubt that in heavy drinkers high blood pressure is very common. Part of the reason may be that many heavy drinkers are overweight. Medical research has shown that if volunteers with normal blood pressures are asked to drink alcohol, their blood pressures go up quickly and then fall quickly. Exactly why alcohol raises blood pressure is not known, but it may have a direct narrowing effect on arteries, increasing the tone in the circulation, and it is possibly also related to stimulation of the sympathetic nervous system and increased levels of adrenaline in the blood. We also know that hypertensives who reduce their alcohol intake may experience a fall in their blood pressures, and certainly alcohol reduction is part of the holistic approach to treating high blood pressure.

On the subject of weight, it is an accepted wisdom that high blood pressure is more common in overweight people than in thin ones. Using undersized blood pressure cuffs can lead to an overestimation of blood pressure in people with large arms, but even if a correct cuff is used, the relationship between obesity and high blood pressure does hold firm. The mechanism is not certain, but it may have something to do with salt intake as well. However, it is unlikely to be as simple as that, and there is much interest now in the role of insulin.

Insulin is a hormone produced by an organ in the abdomen called the pancreas. Insulin regulates blood sugar levels. Failure to produce insulin, or the body's resistance to the blood sugar-lowering effects of insulin, produces diabetes. It has recently been demonstrated that many overweight people are resistant to insulin, and insulin resistance may make people retain salt and water, and hence elevate blood pressure. We know that overweight people may have high blood sugar levels as well as high blood pressure, and it is an intriguing possibility that if insulin resistance could be overcome, then high blood pressure would be less of a problem in overweight people.

On an encouraging note, weight loss does lead to lower blood pressure!

Smoking

The relationship between smoking and hypertension is not, in fact, all that strong. Smoking a cigarette may make the blood pressure go up for a while, but smokers who stop smoking may in fact experience a rise in blood pressure. This is possibly due to the stress of nicotine withdrawal or to the fact that people who have quit smoking may gain weight and eat more salty foods. If you are a hypertensive who has given up smoking, please do not take this as an encouragement to restart, because if you were a hypertensive smoker you would have two risk factors instead of one for heart attacks and strokes.

Diet and Exercise

There are one or two other dietary matters to discuss. For reasons that are totally unclear, vegetarians may have lower blood pressures than meat eaters even after correcting for the difference in salt intake. Coffee intake is also linked to high blood pressure, although cigarette smoking and a high salt diet may accompany high coffee intake, which can make any direct relationship between caffeine and high blood pressure hard to determine. Epidemiologists are still puzzling over this one, but avoiding coffee for a few weeks may lead to a slight lowering of blood pressure.

Exercise is generally considered good for people with high blood pressure. We know that exercise such as running on a treadmill or cycling raises blood pressure, while weightlifting raises blood pressure even more. However, in the long term those who exercise regularly tend to be healthier and have better diets and a lower salt intake than couch potatoes. Even allowing for the fact that people who exercise tend to be more health conscious than their sedentary counterparts, regular exercise does seem to lower blood pressure independently from other factors such as diet.

Before we come to some of the hormonal and biochemical mechanisms that elevate blood pressure, I could not leave out the buzzword that is currently held to be responsible for so many medical conditions - stress! Is there anybody you know, apart from a very few fortunate people who don't have anything to worry about, who does not claim to be stressed? Stress is said to be responsible for everything from dandruff, acne, headaches, constipation and diarrhoea to insomnia, fatigue, palpitations and anti-social behaviour. I do not know anyone doing a challenging job who is not tired and stressed. Of course the pressures of modern life make us stressed, but whereas acute stress, such as a car accident, bereavement or the receipt of a large tax bill can elevate your blood pressure in the short term, there is doubt as to whether a chronically stressful existence actually raises blood pressure. It is of course possible that the stressed-out individual may smoke and drink to excess, eat a diet consisting of too much animal fat and salt and too many calories, and not take any exercise. It is true that a raised blood pressure in association with an acute stressful episode can perhaps be eased by lying in a quiet room listening to whale noises, but patients taking blood pressure pills who blame their entire condition on stress are probably deluding themselves.

Having said that, there are claims that meditation can lower blood pressure in some people, although the mechanism behind this may be more complex than just 'de-stressing'.

Now we move on to glands, organs, hormones and chemicals.

Chapter Three

Mechanisms of High Blood Pressure

First, a piece of revision. Remember that the degree of constriction or relaxation (tone) of the small arterioles largely dictates the pressure inside the circulation. Tone is mediated by small muscle cells that lie in the wall of the arterioles. When the muscle cells contract, the arterioles become narrower, and when they relax, the arterioles dilate. There may well be a vicious circle at play, so that increased pressure inside the arterioles leads to them becoming thicker and more muscular. This in turn reduces their diameter, which in turn leads to pressure going up even further and so on.

There are a whole host of mechanisms in the body that regulate constriction or relaxation of the arterioles. They have the capacity to regulate flow within themselves; this phenomenon (auto-regulation) allows the blood vessels to constrict to reduce the flow through them and to dilate to increase it. This auto-regulation may well be dependent on chemicals produced by the innermost lining of the artery. Nitric oxide is one of the most powerful of these chemicals.

The arterioles are also under the control of the sympathetic nervous system. This is the part of the nervous system that is not under your voluntary control. Tiny sympathetic nerves supply the arterioles. The sympathetic nervous system differs from nerves that can control muscles in our arms and legs. While these can be consciously controlled to produce voluntary contractions of muscles, the sympathetic nervous system can be thought of as the backup mechanism which enables our bodies to react in the most appropriate way to changes in environmental circumstances. The most common of these is the so-called 'fight or flight' reaction, where you react to a stressful situation with stimulation of the sympathetic nervous system to produce a rise in heart rate and blood pressure.

In the wild, the sympathetic nervous system will help a gazelle run away from a lion, but in humans it is the activation of the sympathetic nervous system that gives us sweaty palms and palpitations when we are about to take an exam, or makes our hearts pound when a rogue driver nearly causes a crash on the roads. It is the sympathetic nervous system that protects us by constricting arterioles to less vital areas of the body if we lose blood. *Adrenaline* is the chemical that constricts the vessels. Some people have suggested that overactivity of the sympathetic nervous system is one of the major causes of raised blood pressure. Although it may be responsible for short-lived rises in blood pressure during exercise or when we are under extreme stress, it is probably not responsible for chronically raised blood pressure.

Of equal importance are the renin angiotensin system and the angiotensin- converting enzymes known as ACE. As described in Chapter Two, angiotensin II is a powerful constrictor of arterioles, and it causes aldosterone to be released so that the body retains salt and water. Both these mechanisms raise blood pressure. It is probable that the finger of blame can be pointed at the kidneys. After all, it is the kidneys that control how much salt and water we retain or excrete, and it is the kidneys that produce renin.

There is some experimental evidence to support this. For these experiments we owe a debt of gratitude to a special breed of rat with genetically determined hypertension. Kidneys from such hypertensive rats were transplanted into normal rats, and the normal rats developed high blood pressure. Similarly, taking a kidney from a normal rat and transplanting it into one of the hypertensive rats led to the hypertensive rat's blood pressure becoming normal. Common sense and medical ethics prevent us from carrying out such Frankenstein-like experiments on humans. There is some circumstantial evidence in humans, however, as patients who have had kidney failure due to high blood pressure may end up with normal blood pressures after a successful kidney transplant.

There are other hormones and chemicals which contribute to regulating the pressure in the blood vessels, but they are probably less important than the ones I have already described.

Primary and Secondary Hypertension

All these mechanisms may contribute to the condition of 'Essential Hypertension'. This is a really confusing term, as most of us regard the word 'essential' as being equivalent to necessary, but what it actually means is primary hypertension with a complicated chemical and genetic basis that can be treated but not cured. Ninety five per cent of people with hypertension have essential or primary hypertension.

Secondary hypertension occurs when there is a specific condition which, when treated, often leads to the blood pressure returning to normal. Some drugs can also induce secondary hypertension.

The Adrenal Glands and Pituitary Gland

I have talked about the kidneys as the source of high blood pressure, but above each kidney is a small gland called the adrenal gland, and occasionally the malfunction of these glands can cause high blood pressure. Both adrenal glands can sometimes be overactive, or there can be a small tumour in one of the glands, called an *adenoma*. Either of these abnormalities - overactivity or a tumour - can lead to an overproduction of the hormone aldosterone, leading to salt- and water-retention and raised blood pressure. The condition that results when the body manufactures too much aldosterone for its own good is often called Conn's Syndrome. Sometimes this is associated with low potassium in the blood, because aldosterone makes the body retain salt at the expense of losing potassium.

Another glandular condition associated with high blood pressure is called Cushing's Syndrome, which results in overproduction of a hormone called cortisol. This can be due to an abnormality of either the adrenal gland or the pituitary gland in the brain. The pituitary gland produces hormones to control the activity of other glands around the body, including the thyroid and the adrenals. When the body produces too much cortisol, sufferers may develop typical symptoms such as a moon-shaped face, central obesity (weight gained around the middle rather than on the hips or elsewhere on the body), skin streaks like stretch marks called *striae*, thinning of the bones (which may lead to fractures), raised blood sugar and high blood pressure. Treating the condition by removing the abnormal gland (either the pituitary or the adrenal gland) will usually return the blood pressure to normal.

A rare kind of tumour of the adrenal gland leads to overproduction of adrenaline or its related chemical, noradrenaline. This overproduction can be intermittent or continuous, and the symptoms can be quite dramatic. Surges of blood pressure may occur in response to the production of adrenaline, along with symptoms such as rapid palpitations due to a fast heart rate and marked hot flushes and sweating. Sometimes the huge surges in blood pressure can actually lead to heart attacks or strokes. These tumours (see Chapter Six) are called phaeochromocytomas, this is often shortened to phaeo (pronounced fee-o).

A different sort of pituitary tumour in the brain can lead to overproduction of growth hormone, the hormone that makes us grow normally. In people with a condition known as acromegaly, the bones in the hands, feet and the skull may grow and grow, producing the characteristic appearance of a jutting jaw, abnormally large hands and feet, and enlargement of organs such as the tongue and the heart. High blood pressure occurs commonly in these people; once again, removal of the tumour will usually return the blood pressure to normal.

Conditions Affecting the Arterial Tree

There are two specific conditions affecting the arterial tree that can directly cause high blood pressure. One of these is called 'coarctation of the aorta', where the person is born with an hour-glass-shaped narrowing in the aorta in the chest. This condition can cause high blood pressure in childhood, although in some cases it may not be discovered until later in life. It is often associated with an abnormality of one of the heart valves and produces a delay in the appearance of the pulses in the feet compared to the pulses at the wrist. It also produces characteristic changes on a chest x-ray. Coarctation can sometimes be seen on a cardiac ultrasound, or more often by more modern x-ray techniques, such as CT scanning or by MRI (Magnetic Resonance Imaging). Coarctations may be repaired surgically or by a procedure in which the narrowing is dilated with a balloon.

The other arterial abnormality involves a narrowing of one or both of the renal arteries as they arise from the aorta. The renal arteries supply the kidneys with blood. Renal artery narrowings can occur in older people as part of the general process of hardening or furring up of the arteries. After all, there is no reason why the kidney arteries should not become narrowed in the same way that the coronary arteries to the heart or the carotid arteries to the brain become narrowed. However, in younger people below the age of 40, this 'renal artery stenosis' may be the result of a specific condition. We believe that the reason this is associated with high blood pressure is that these narrowings can reduce the blood flow to the kidneys, thus mimicking a situation where blood pressure is low because of blood loss. This stimulates the kidneys to produce renin in order to try and conserve salt and water.

Kidney Disease

Diabetes is one of the most common medical conditions to affect the kidneys, but nearly all diseases that lead to chronic kidney damage can cause high blood pressure. Inflammation of the kidneys produces a condition called 'glomerulonephritis'. This may lead to progressive worsening of kidney function, and be associated with high blood pressure. There are a variety of causes of such inflammation, but some people with this condition may end up on kidney machines to purify the blood (dialysis). Sometimes a kidney transplant is needed.

'Polycystic kidneys' is a condition where the kidneys develop abnormally and contain several cysts. This condition can be associated with abnormal arterial swellings in the brain, called aneurysms. People with this condition may have high blood pressure and also may suffer brain haemorrhages.

Drugs and Hypertension

Many drugs can raise blood pressure, either directly or indirectly. For example, any drugs that damage the kidneys irreversibly (such as certain antibiotics given in very high doses) can cause hypertension. Some nasal decongestants and even slimming pills contain chemicals that mimic the action of adrenaline and can raise blood pressure. Cyclosporin, a powerful drug for preventing rejection of transplanted organs, can also raise blood pressure.

Probably the most common drugs associated with high blood pressure nowadays are the contraceptive pill and hormone replacement therapy (HRT). The more modern pills with a lower dose of oestrogen may be less blameworthy than the old-fashioned ones, and pills that contain only progesterone probably do not raise blood pressure.

It is important for any woman starting on the contraceptive pill to remember that careful monitoring of blood pressure is absolutely crucial, and if her blood pressure does go up on the pill, then serious consideration should be given to taking a different sort of pill or stopping it altogether. Doctors would normally recommend that any woman taking the pill should have her blood pressure checked at least once a year, and probably more frequently - up to three or four times a year if she is over the age of 30. Obviously the decision to carry on or stop taking the pill will be one that should be discussed with a woman's GP or gynaecologist. The risks and benefits of carrying on with the pill or changing to another form of contraception must be weighed up for each individual person.

There has been much debate about whether women with hypertension should take HRT, and whether HRT actually causes hypertension or not. Some women will gain weight and retain salt and water with hormone replacement therapy, and this may have an effect in raising blood pressure. The current thinking is that HRT does not actually raise blood pressure directly, and that mild elevations in blood pressure should not deter women from taking HRT if it is thought necessary. HRT has until very recently had some very good publicity in terms of reducing the risk of heart attacks and strokes, although its benefits have never been fully proven. Recently one particular form of HRT has had some bad publicity as heart attacks and strokes were more common in women taking this preparation. Obviously there are other factors, such as a family history of breast cancer, which may deter women from taking HRT. Current thinking again would suggest that even if women are on treatment for high blood pressure they should not be denied the benefits of HRT if there are good reasons for taking it (see Chapter Nine).

I will end this chapter by mentioning the peculiarly named 'White Coat Hypertension'. I say 'peculiarly' because few doctors actually wear white coats these days! In any case, this term describes the high blood pressure that occurs only when someone has to visit a doctor or hospital. The theory is that some people are so anxious about having their blood pressure taken that their blood pressure goes up whenever they have to have it measured. Doctors often see this with their own eyes, because when they approach the patient with the blood pressure cuff, it causes the patient to flush and his or her pulse rate to shoot up. While doctors will always try to put such people at ease, in some cases their blood pressure, even if taken three or four times, may not settle until they leave the clinic or hospital. Sometimes it is useful for the blood pressure reading to be taken in the person's home, or assessed on a 24-hour blood pressure monitor (see Chapter Six).

Even if sufferers from 'white coat hypertension' are not prescribed blood pressure pills straight away, they need to be carefully observed, as there is some evidence to suggest that it is only a matter of time before sustained elevations of blood pressure develop.

Chapter Four

How Is High Blood Pressure Diagnosed?

According to some of the older medical text books, and the many popular magazines that claim to make the public more health-conscious, high blood pressure always causes headaches, nose bleeds, spots in front of the eyes and a pounding in the head. It is also alleged to make people tired. What is striking in clinical practice is just how unusual these symptoms are, with the exception of tiredness. It seems that virtually everybody is tired; this is probably a reflection of the fact that in the United Kingdom we work longer hours than most of our European counterparts. Tiredness is not a specific symptom of high blood pressure but, of course, if you go to your GP complaining of tiredness and you leave the surgery without having had your blood pressure taken, then I am afraid that your GP is failing in his or her duty to you. The fact is that the vast majority of people with high blood pressure do not have any symptoms at all, and hypertension may first come to light completely by accident.

Many people going to their GPs complaining of indigestion or a skin rash, for example, will hopefully have their blood pressure taken, which can start the ball rolling. Other people may attend a medical for life insurance or for pre-employment purposes, or even go to one of the many Well Man or Well Woman clinics which are now available. Sometimes people check their blood pressure at the local chemist's shop and find it is high. I saw a patient recently who, while visiting his in-laws, had a go on his father-in-law's new blood pressure machine and found that his blood pressure reading came out as elevated.

These people who have high blood pressure picked up totally by accident should regard themselves as extremely fortunate. Those less lucky may have hypertension diagnosed only after the occurrence of a complication, for example a heart attack, a major or minor stroke, or a cardiac rhythm disturbance.

Sadly, even today hypertension is severely underdiagnosed. Doctors in the United States and the United Kingdom have coined the phrase 'the rule of halves'. This means that in ordinary medical practice only half of all patients with high blood pressure will be correctly diagnosed, and only half of those will receive anti-hypertensive treatment. Of these, only half of those will have their blood pressure well controlled. Thus, only about 12.5 per cent, or one patient in eight with high blood pressure, actually receives the correct treatment.

It is not just hypertension that is neglected in this way. Similar studies have shown that unless the medical profession makes a huge effort, we are not as good as we should be at identifying people with elevated cholesterol levels. A study from the United States showed that only half of the patients who underwent heart operations had had their cholesterol levels measured, and only a small percentage of those actually received appropriate cholesterol-lowering drugs.

Treating high blood pressure saves lives, although it is always difficult to know precisely how many lives could be saved if high blood pressure were treated with appropriate rigour. It is estimated that about 300 people in the United Kingdom die from the complications of high blood pressure every six weeks. In a pithy analogy, Drs Beevers and Macgregor have likened this to a jumbo jet crashing every six weeks, killing all passengers. They have pointed out, quite rightly, that this would produce public outrage and a massive action to improve air safety. Is it acceptable for 300 patients with hypertension to die unnecessarily every six weeks? Of course not. It is scandalous.

It is both a failure of medical education and a lack of awareness of the dangers associated with even mild elevations of high blood pressure that have led to this rather laissez-faire attitude to the treatment of hypertension. I see many patients with levels of blood pressure that are clearly above normal who have had their blood pressures 'monitored' for a period of years. To be quite honest, I am not sure what the purpose of watching and monitoring high blood pressure is. If a patient presents with a breast lump or has an abnormal shadow picked up on a chest x-ray, doctors leap into action and treatment is started. We do not watch or monitor breast lumps or lung tumours!

Individuals concerned with trying to raise awareness of health issues in the general public have quite rightly pointed out the importance of self-examination for breast lumps, the importance of regular cervical smears, and have tried quite correctly to raise the awareness of testicular and prostate cancer in males. Cancer is a dramatic illness that can kill people quickly, and it captures the public imagination. Hypertension, unfortunately, is a poor relation grabbing less interest from politicians, and it is not a particularly sexy subject for the health pages of our newspapers. This really is a tragedy. There are so many people walking around with mild to moderate elevations in blood pressure whose prospect of good health in the future could be greatly enhanced by having their blood pressure treated and avoiding the often catastrophic complications.

In the UK, the government's National Service Framework (NSF) for coronary heart disease has started to ensure that the need to treat high blood pressure is firmly etched in the minds of general practitioners and primary care organisations. One of the catch phrases in the NSF is that 'excellence means doing the simple things correctly all the time' - and this means checking blood pressure, prescribing medication appropriately and checking that the tablets are working! This applies not just to people who have had heart attacks and strokes, but to those who haven't, just to ensure things stay that way.

I described earlier how doctors make the measurements of systolic and diastolic blood pressure. Although many experts recommend that ideally the patient should be seated, in hospitals it is often done with the patient lying down on a couch. It is a good idea for the blood pressure be measured at least twice, especially on initial consultations when the person may be unfamiliar with the doctor and with the discomfort of having the cuff pumped up around the arm. Some consideration must also be given to whether they have just dashed into the surgery with a red face, huffing and puffing, or whether the patient has been seated relaxed in the waiting room for a while. It is generally recommended that the second of the two readings is taken as the more accurate.

Patients may find that there is a discrepancy in the readings obtained at their GP's surgery compared with readings obtained by a nurse in the Occupational Health Department at work or by a consultant or other hospital doctor. These differences may reflect the levels of comfort or anxiety of the patient, but unfortunately some of the errors may be due to the fact that not everybody is trained in how to take a blood pressure reading correctly.

Surveys have shown that not everybody obeys the exact rules about the appearance and disappearance of the pulse sounds. This probably reflects the fact that some people are taught to measure blood pressure by experienced doctors, while others may have learned in a more academic environment, at medical school, and have not had training continued at a later date.

Another cause for the discrepancy is the use of automatic electronic machines which print out numbers in bright red digits and which involve very little input from the physician or nurse taking the blood pressure! It is wise to maintain a healthy scepticism about the accuracy of these machines. Please remember that just because a machine prints out a number in bright red digits it does not mean it is accurate; there are some machines that are reliable, and which have been tested and found to be accurate, but this cannot be said for all of them. If you have a machine, it is a good idea to check its accuracy against a standard traditional mercury manometer.

If your GP thinks your blood pressure is high, he or she may well shine a light into your eyes - this is to look at the blood vessels in the retina at the back of your eyes. Long-standing high blood pressure can cause changes in the arteries and veins in the retina; the presence of such changes might give your GP an idea of whether you have had raised blood pressure for a long time.

Often, because of the worry about committing patients to treatment on the basis of one or two readings in a doctor's surgery, many doctors are now employing a 24-hour ambulatory blood pressure monitor. This is an intrusive device, as many people who have had one fitted can testify. Essentially, it means wearing a blood pressure cuff attached to a machine that pumps the cuff up automatically several times during the day and night. This checks what your blood pressure is doing in your own environment, rather than in the artificial surroundings of a doctor's surgery. Although some blood pressure experts are sceptical about the use of a 24-hour blood pressure monitor, my own view is that it is a very useful clinical tool. It allows doctors to weed out patients who have 'white coat hypertension'. But even if the readings are consistently abnormal, they may be less stratospheric than the readings obtained in the doctor's surgery. This can guide the doctor towards starting treatment with gentler medication and at lower doses than might have been the case if the doctor relied only on the measurement obtained in the surgery. Your doctor can also see from a blood pressure monitor whether the readings go up during particularly stressful times of the day - it is sometimes possible to tailor specific drug therapy depending on what the monitor shows.

If after reading so far you are curious about why the medical profession is (or at least should be) so obsessed with high blood pressure, then please read on. But a word of warning: the next chapter is not for the squeamish!

Chapter Five

Why Is High Blood Pressure So Dangerous?

Let's not beat about the bush - hypertension is one of the most common, if not *the* most common, risk factor for vascular disease in Western populations. Some rather old data from the late 1950s shows that patients with a diastolic blood pressure of between 110 and 130 had an 80 per cent chance of surviving two years. This may not sound too bad, but put another way, it means that one in five of these patients will die within two years, which is pretty awful.

Do remember that these statistics were obtained long before the newer treatments for blood pressure were available. With effective treatment, death rates have, of course, dropped. However, before you can have it treated you have to have it diagnosed, and following the rule of halves described in Chapter Four, there are many people walking around with blood pressures at this level who do not know about it. There is no reason to believe that 21st-century people with diastolic pressures of between 110 and 130 on no treatment will do any better than their predecessors of 50 years ago. Doctors are often accused of being harbingers of doom and gloom, especially by patients who may have a cavalier attitude to their illnesses. However, they have a duty to point out the facts, and most people would agree that giving yourself a one-in-five chance of dying within two years by not following medical advice is not sensible.

Even with milder elevations such as diastolic pressures of between 95 and 105, the annual death rate for a person in their mid-40s is three times greater than in patients of a similar age with normal pressures. To put it bluntly, data from a large insurance company in the early 1960s showed that a 35-year-old man with a blood pressure of 150/100 had only a 50:50 chance of surviving to the age of 60 unless his blood pressure was treated! Old data that may be, but there is no reason to suppose that not treating high blood pressure now has any better outcome than it did then.

The scale of the problem is huge in terms of the actual numbers of patients affected. Milder grades of hypertension are more common than severe grades, and diastolic pressures between 90 and 110 are found in about 20 per cent of middle-aged adults. It is less common in the young and more common in the elderly: roughly 50 per cent of people aged 70 or more will have a blood pressure of 160/95 or higher at a one-off reading in the doctor's surgery. We can estimate that approximately 15 per cent of the entire population of England and Wales will have blood pressures like this, and that an average GP might have around 300 patients on his or her list with readings of 160/95 or more.

In the United States, blood pressures of this level have been estimated to affect twenty-three million people! This represents between 15 and 20 per cent of white people and up to 30 per cent of people of African and Caribbean origin between the ages of 18 and 74. This is a staggeringly large number of people who are deemed otherwise healthy and yet who are walking around with a potentially lethal risk factor for becoming a heart attack or stroke statistic.

Complications

Although the absolute risk of any individual with a diastolic reading of 95-105 dying prematurely within five years is small, there is still the risk of other complications.

The complications of high blood pressure can be disastrous. The high pressure within the vascular tree leads to a condition known as 'end organ damage'. Various organs, particularly the heart, the brain and the kidneys, can be damaged, and more often than not this damage is due to disease occurring in the blood vessels which supply those organs. I mentioned earlier about the resistance in the arterioles being raised, and as a consequence of this the arterioles becoming thickened as the smooth muscle cells in the walls of the arterioles multiply. Until recently we believed that the vessels became thickened as a passive reaction to high blood pressure, but modern research has suggested that high blood pressure and thickening of blood vessels may both be part of the same disease. Earlier in this book I described angiotensin-converting enzyme, or ACE, which circulates around in the blood. However, ACE also exists within the tissues, and abnormally high levels of ACE in the tissues

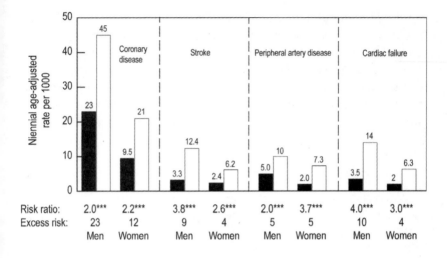

Figure 5.1

Graph from the Framingham study, showing the increased risk of vascular disease and heart failure in those with high blood pressure over a 30-year period. The black columns show the risk in those with normal pressures, and the white bars the risk in high blood pressure. The risk for men and women between the ages of 35 and 64 years of age are shown separately. The 'risk-ratio' underneath quantifies the risk - so, for example, hypertensive men are 3.8 times as likely to have a stroke as men with normal pressure, and 4 times as likely to develop heart failure.

From European Heart Journal *1992, by permission*

may stimulate the development of muscle thickening. As the muscles thicken it is often at the expense of the diameter of the blood vessels and, as this becomes further reduced, so the resistance to flow increases even more.

Hypertension is one of the most common causes of hardening of the arteries, often known as *arteriosclerosis*. At the same time as the muscle coat of the artery thickens, the lining of the artery becomes damaged and fatty deposits called *atheroma* develop in the arterial tree. The fact that many hypertensive people also have raised cholesterol, are smokers or have diabetes only compounds the tendency to arterial injury.

One of the largest epidemiological studies ever done looked at the incidence of heart disease, strokes and peripheral vascular disease in a town called Framingham in the United States. The population was followed up for several years to see what happened to them. Figure 5.1 shows the incidence of vascular disease in men and women under the age of 65 with high blood pressure compared to those with normal pressure, over three decades. In both sexes there was a 200

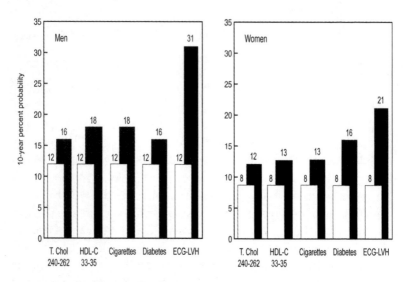

Risk of coronary disease in hypertension and associated risk factors. Subjects aged 52-54 years in the Framingham Study. □ = high blood pressure alone (160-172); ■ = associated risk factor; T. Chol = total cholesterol; HDL-C = high density cholesterol.

Figure 5.2

This graph shows how the presence of other risk factors such as high cholesterol, cigarette smoking and diabetes increase the probability of developing heart disease in patients with high blood pressure. The white bars show patients with high blood pressure alone, the black bars show those with the other risk factors. The right-hand column shows how thickening of the heart muscle (ECG-LVH) also compounds the risk of developing coronary artery disease in both men and women.

From European Heart Journal *1992, by permission*

to 400 per cent increase in risk! Another striking result of this observational study was the finding that if patients with high blood pressure had other risk factors such as smoking, diabetes or raised cholesterol, then the risk of developing coronary artery disease was much higher (Figure 5.2).

Thickened Heart Muscle

What exactly does high blood pressure do to the heart? One of the first abnormalities is that the heart muscle becomes thickened. Basically a heart that has to work in a high-pressure system is, in fact, 'pumping iron'. In the same way that the biceps or chest muscles can be made to develop at the gym by using machines that make the muscles work against high resistance, so the heart muscle thickens when it has to pump blood in a high-pressure circulation. The heart is 'working out'! There is quite a close relationship between the height of the blood pressure and the degree of thickening of the heart muscle. The condition of the heart muscle thickening is known as *left ventricular hypertrophy*, often abbreviated to LVH. However, we now believe that elevations of the ACE levels in the tissue might contribute directly to thickening of the heart muscle as well.

Sometimes thickening of the heart muscle can be detected on a clinical examination, but more often than not it is picked up on the heartbeat trace known as the electrocardiogram or ECG. It may also be seen on a cardiac ultrasound examination.

There is some evidence that having a thick heart muscle due to high blood pressure increases the chance of having a heart attack, and a higher incidence of developing heart failure in future years. (See Fig. 5.2). If the blood pressure is not lowered, then eventually this thickened, overworked heart will become tired and start beating less strongly. This can produce heart failure, where the person may be short of breath, tired and prone to serious rhythm disturbances which can sometimes be fatal. People with heart failure are often partially or totally disabled and dependent on an array of tablets to keep them out of hospital.

Recently we have recognised another sort of heart failure that can develop when the heart muscle is thickened. This is where the heart may not only contract inadequately but also relax poorly. Normally when the heart muscle relaxes between beats, the pressure inside the main pumping chambers falls down very rapidly to normal, but when

43

the heart muscle is thickened it may be stiff and inelastic and the pressures may remain high. This can also cause the same symptoms of fatigue and breathlessness. Both these forms of heart failure can be prevented in many people through good blood pressure control.

Narrowing of the Arteries and Angina

It is well known that furring-up of the coronary arteries is common in people with high blood pressure. In fact, it is twice as common in hypertensive people as in the rest of the population. Again, the higher the blood pressure, the greater the risk of a heart attack. It is estimated that about 1 per cent of people with high blood pressure suffer a full-blown heart attack each year; this may rise to 3 per cent where the blood pressure is not well controlled, and even higher if there are other risk factors such as smoking or diabetes.

If the coronary arteries become furred-up and narrowed, then the heart muscle starts to become deprived of oxygen. This is because the coronary arteries are essentially the fuel pipes that deliver oxygen into the heart muscle. Under normal circumstances when the coronary arteries are healthy, even the demands made by the heart muscle during vigorous exercise can be met by an adequate blood supply. If the arteries are narrowed, however, they cannot meet this extra demand, and then the heart muscle may develop cramp on exercise. This is the condition known as angina.

Heart Attack (Myocardial Infarction)

Although many people with hypertension may have angina, some will have a heart attack (known as a *myocardial infarction*) out of the blue. This occurs when a blood clot suddenly blocks off an artery, and part of the heart muscle dies. This of course may be fatal. High blood pressure inside an artery may impose abnormal stresses and strains on the areas where deposits of cholesterol have occurred, and this may in turn cause blood clots to form.

Recent research has shown how dangerous high blood pressure can be. Many heart attacks, some fatal, occur within a few hours of waking up in the mornings. Figure 5.3 shows the results of a study published in 1994. The largest number of heart attacks occurred in the first few hours after waking up. Similarly, another study from 1992

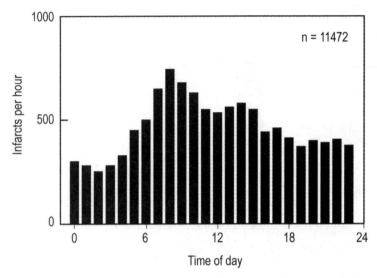

Time of onset of acute myocardial infarction in total study population.

Figure 5.3

Graph showing the time of day at which heart attacks occur. The highest incidence occurs in the hours after awakening.
From European Heart Journal *1994, by permission*

showed that sudden cardiac death occurs most frequently at these times (Figure 5.4). The surges of blood pressure that occur at this time may be at least partly responsible for imposing stresses and strains on the coronary arteries and promoting the formation of blood clots. The blood pressure recording (Figure 5.5) shows a real example of this. Before 6.00 a.m. both systolic and diastolic readings shot up in this patient. The actual readings went from 127/74 to 194/114 in the space of half an hour. This patient's high blood pressure was picked up after he suffered a small stroke whilst driving.

One of these studies showed that heart attacks were particularly likely to occur on Mondays (Figure 5.6) giving rise to the phrase 'Mondays are bad for your heart'! Many of us recognise the gloom that Monday mornings bring, but the message for patients with hypertension is that although your heart may sink as the alarm goes off on Monday morning, your blood pressure probably does not!

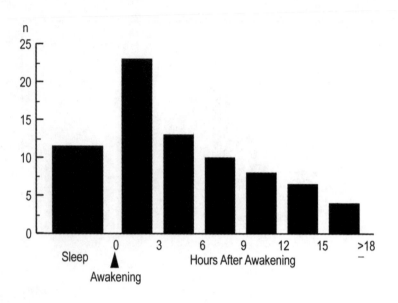

Figure 5.4
Graph showing the time of day at which sudden death occurs in relation to the time of waking up. The most frequent time is within the first three hours after waking up.
From American Journal of Cardiology *1992, by permission*

Joking aside, this research has stimulated the pharmaceutical industry to produce medications that provide twenty four hour blood pressure control and avoid these surges.

The government's National Service Framework document quite correctly states that all patients who have had a heart attack should have their blood pressures treated and lowered to the recommended levels, or as close to these levels as humanly possible.

It is worth mentioning here that cardiologists will see quite a few hypertensive patients with chest pains, and that many of these patients will turn out to have nothing wrong with their arteries at all. There is a theory that when the heart muscle thickens in hypertensive patients, the blood supply to the heart muscle cannot keep up and so this thickened heart muscle is short of blood. This may explain why when cardiologists investigate patients with chest pains and high blood pressure, they often find that the coronary arteries look normal. However, it would be irresponsible of a doctor

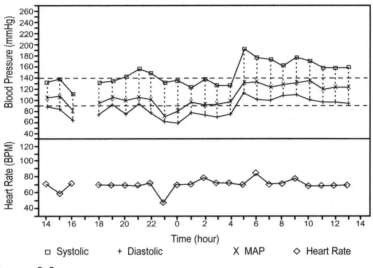

Figure 5.5

24-hour blood pressure monitor from patient who had suffered a small stroke while driving. Note the large surge in both systolic and diastolic pressures before 6 a.m. Such surges in pressure may contribute to heart attacks, strokes and sudden death in the first few hours after awakening.

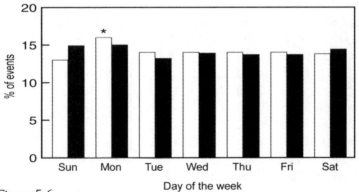

Figure 5.6

Graph showing the weekly distribution of heart attacks in non-smokers (hatched bars) and smokers (black bars). The asterisk indicates a statistically higher incidence on Mondays.

From European Heart Journal *1994, by permission*

to assume that angina-like chest pain in a patient with high blood pressure was due to a mismatch between the muscle and its blood supply rather than to an actual narrowing of one or more coronary arteries. A good doctor will make a clinical judgement about how far to take investigations in any patient, and this will often depend on how the doctor judges the overall coronary risk. I will give more information on this later in the book.

Heart Failure

If the heart becomes damaged by one or more heart attacks, then this can also increase the likelihood of heart failure developing. This is independent of the heart muscle becoming worn out and fatigued from many years of pumping against a high pressure.

Heart failure is four times more common in hypertensive women, and seven times more common in hypertensive men, than in groups of similar ages with normal pressures.

Atrial Fibrillation

The other common complication affecting the heart is a rhythm disturbance called atrial fibrillation, often abbreviated to AF. This is a condition where the upper chambers of the heart (atria) stop beating regularly. Instead they shiver and shake, generating haphazard electrical impulses at a frequency of about 600 per minute. The lower pumping chambers (ventricles) receive far too many messages to beat, and they respond much too fast and irregularly. This may produce uncomfortable, rapid palpitations. It is not at all uncommon for high blood pressure to be diagnosed for the first time in patients who go to their doctors with the symptoms of atrial fibrillation. High blood pressure is probably the most common identifiable cause of atrial fibrillation in the Western world. However, not all patients with atrial fibrillation will notice it, and sometimes this is also picked up at a routine examination.

Atrial fibrillation has two possible disastrous consequences. First, because the atria are not beating properly, blood clots can form inside them. These can then break off and travel round the circulation and get stuck in another artery. These travelling clots are known as *emboli*. Unfortunately the most common place for them to go is the brain, where they can cause minor or major strokes, depending upon the size of the clot. Small emboli may cause transient symptoms such as difficulty speaking, loss of vision in one eye, or weakness on one side of the body, but the symptoms may disappear within minutes or a few hours. These are mini-strokes, properly called *transient ischaemic attacks*, often abbreviated to TIAs. Anybody experiencing such symptoms should consult their doctor immediately, as they can be warnings of a major stroke to come.

Emboli can also travel to any other artery such as to the arm or leg, or even into one of the arteries supplying the intestines. The second disaster is that if the heart is allowed to beat too fast for too long it can enlarge and weaken and, again, cause heart failure. Drugs can be used to slow the heart down. Patients with atrial fibrillation are nearly always advised to take aspirin or Warfarin to thin the blood and to reduce the risk of clots breaking off and causing emboli. It is often possible to convert the heart back to a normal rhythm using an electric shock given under a short general anaesthetic. It then may be necessary to take medication to stop the fibrillation recurring.

However, sometimes it is not possible to switch the upper chambers back to a normal rhythm. Patients with hypertension should not regard this as an unmitigated disaster. There are millions of people walking around the planet quite happily with atrial fibrillation and, so long as medications are taken to stop the heart racing and to protect against strokes, then there should be no restrictions at all on activity.

Warfarin
Many will know that Warfarin is rat poison and people are, therefore, reluctant to take it. Let me reassure you that Warfarin in the therapeutic dose used by doctors has been around for many years. It can be taken quite safely as long as the required dose is controlled by regular blood tests to make sure that the blood is not too thin, which would put you at risk of bleeding, and not too thick in which case there would be a continued risk of strokes. It is a bit inconvenient to have blood tests three or four times a week when Warfarin is commenced, but once the dose is stabilised then blood tests become less frequent, maybe only three or four times a year.

Certain drugs, particularly antibiotics, may interfere with Warfarin, and so a temporary adjustment of the dose may be needed by the anti-coagulant clinic which is controlling your medication. For some reason it is a common misconception that Warfarin and alcohol cannot be taken together. This is just not the case. It is quite reasonable to take moderate regular amounts of alcohol with Warfarin, but what you should *not* do is to drink nothing for four or five days and then to binge-drink and get pie-eyed. This can play havoc with the blood clotting. Warfarin is broken down by the liver, and if your liver takes a hammering with alcohol, then Warfarin is not metabolised so efficiently, the blood becomes too thin, and bleeding might occur. On the other hand, a steady and moderate consumption of alcohol is perfectly easy for anti-coagulant clinics to cope with.

Patients on Warfarin will normally carry a small book around with their dose requirements tabled for them, and the three letters 'INR'. This stands for International Normalised Ratio and is a reflection of how thin your blood is compared to blood from people not taking Warfarin. Therefore, an INR of 1 means that the blood is not thinned at all, whereas an INR of 2 means that it is twice as thin as normal. In people with fibrillation, doctors like to keep the INR at around 2.5.

Not every patient with atrial fibrillation needs to be on Warfarin. However, people with hypertension and who have fibrillation with a thickened heart muscle are at an increased risk of strokes compared to some younger people who may have fibrillation as a primary electrical abnormality, and not as a complication of high blood pressure. These younger people may be all right on aspirin, but hypertensives are probably much better treated with Warfarin. It is a matter of individual clinical judgement, and your doctor should discuss with you whether you should take Warfarin or aspirin, and give you reasons for his or her decision.

Stroke

Although atrial fibrillation can be a cause of strokes, strokes can occur in hypertensive people for other reasons as well. There is no point in mincing words - a stroke can be a disaster, turning an active, able-bodied individual into a wheelchair-bound, paralysed person unable to speak and barely able to fend for him- or herself. Not all strokes are like this, and I may stand accused of being melodramatic, but you only have to go round a stroke rehabilitation unit to see how devastating this condition can be. Strokes are less common than heart attacks in middle-aged people, but strokes are as common as heart attacks in older people with high blood pressure.

Strokes can occur either because of a haemorrhage into the brain or because an artery gets blocked off, causing part of the brain to die in the same way that part of the heart muscle can die. It is a sad indictment of our medical system that people may only be found to be hypertensive once they have had a stroke, and there can be fewer more poignant examples of shutting the stable door after the horse has bolted than prescribing an anti-hypertensive drug *after* a patient has had a stroke rather than before. The early morning surges in blood pressure may be just as responsible for the timing of strokes as for heart attacks (see Figure 5.5).

Immediately after a stroke doctors may be worried about lowering the blood pressure too quickly for fear of further reducing the blood flow into the damaged brain, but in the long term aggressive treatment is necessary. If a person survives a stroke, then controlling blood pressure definitely reduces the chance of having another one. This is fine if the first stroke was a minor one, but may not be so useful if the first stroke was a disabling one.

Transient Ischaemic Attacks
Some people experience mini-strokes, which are properly known, as mentioned above, as *transient ischaemic attacks* (TIAs).

With TIA you may experience some neurological symptoms such as weakness on one side or of one limb, or transient loss of speech or loss of vision in one eye. This may all resolve in a matter of minutes or within a few hours, leaving no permanent deficit. A TIA can be the forerunner of a major stroke, however, and certainly should be investigated.

Population surveys have shown that treating even mild hypertension can be expected to produce approximately a 40 per cent reduction in the incidence of strokes. As strokes are more common in older people, treatment is particularly effective for this group.

Needless to say, if there are other risk factors such as smoking and a high cholesterol level in a hypertensive person, then these must also be addressed.

Subarachnoid Haemorrhage

One particularly devastating and fortunately rarer form of brain complication is called a subarachnoid haemorrhage. This is where blood leaks out into the delicate membranes that line the brain and into the spinal fluid. This often is signalled by a severe headache with loss of consciousness. Some people with this condition may have a small swelling of an artery in the brain, called an *aneurysm*, while others may have the rare condition known as polycystic kidneys (see Chapter Three).

Claudication

Given that people with hypertension may have widespread abnormalities of the arterial tree, it is not uncommon for them to develop problems with the blood flow into the legs as the arteries in the pelvis and the legs can become narrowed or blocked. This can produce a condition called 'claudication' which can affect the calf muscles and even the buttocks. People may get severe pain in these muscles when they walk; treatment by balloon dilation or surgery to the blocked arteries may be necessary. Doctors have to be careful what drugs they use to treat hypertension in these people, because some drugs can constrict the arteries in the legs and make the symptoms of claudication worse (see Chapters Seven and Eight).

One particularly dangerous condition is where the aorta, which is the main artery that leaves the heart, giving off branches all round the body, can become damaged. There are two things that can happen to the aorta. It can either progressively dilate to produce a large swelling (an aneurysm - this occurs particularly commonly in the abdomen), or suffer a dissection (see page 53). Aneurysms may only produce symptoms when they are about to rupture, and if they do rupture it is often fatal. As part of screening hypertensive people, it is useful to do an ultrasound examination of the abdomen, where the aorta can be seen and its diameter measured. If the aorta in the abdomen is more than 6cm wide, then repair of this is recommended and can be carried out at low risk. If we wait until the aneurysm is about to rupture, the operation is much more dangerous. People with dilated aortas that have not yet reached 6cm need to be scanned at regular intervals. Needless to say, they must have their blood pressures controlled rigorously.

Dissection

The second condition that can afflict the aorta is known as a dissection. This is where blood leaks into the weakened wall of the aorta and travels up the wall separating the layers of the aorta, in the same way the two layers of a paper handkerchief may be separated. This again may be a catastrophic condition producing tearing or ripping pain in the back and, if the tear involves some of the branches coming off the aorta, then symptoms such as loss of the pulse in one arm, symptoms of stroke and damage to the kidneys may also occur. Sometimes the dissection damages the main valve that separates the heart from the aorta, causing it to leak. A dissection is often a surgical emergency, but even emergency repair does not guarantee survival.

Some people with dissections of the aorta do not require surgery but need a prolonged period of hospital treatment to lower their blood pressures right down to normal levels.

You will by now have got the picture that high blood pressure is a bad thing for arteries around the body. I hope that anyone who has had doubts about taking their blood pressure pills will have had their doubts completely dispelled!

Kidney Damage

I'm afraid the bad news is not finished yet, however. High blood pressure can damage the kidneys, and there is good evidence that controlling blood pressure can prevent harm to the kidneys over a long period of time. Some people will develop hypertension as a result of chronic kidney disease, but the converse is also true, as people may develop kidney disease as a result of high blood pressure, which can make the kidneys less efficient at removing waste material from the body. People with kidney failure are unwell and anaemic and, once the kidneys are damaged, the ability to take certain medications is limited because they are not excreted efficiently by your body. Some people with kidney failure need to go on to dialysis because the kidneys cannot get rid of salt and water, and without dialysis the body becomes overloaded with fluid. Fluid may accumulate in the tissues - this is known as *oedema* (fluid retention), often affecting the legs. If you press oedema with your thumb, it may leave a dent known as *pitting*. If the lungs become overloaded with oedema fluid, the patient may become very breathless. This can be dangerous because the lungs cannot deliver enough oxygen into the blood, and always requires admission to hospital.

Sometimes a kidney transplant is necessary if the kidney damage is quite severe, but unfortunately, hypertension is common in kidney transplant patients. The reasons why transplant patients develop high blood pressure are very complicated and may be due to an immune reaction. Even some of the drugs used to prevent rejection can themselves cause high blood pressure.

Eye Damage

My last piece of bad news for the organs of the body is for the eyes. The arteries in the eyes can suffer as a result of high blood pressure to varying degrees. Sometimes they just appear slightly thickened, but in more serious cases there can be haemorrhages in the retina at the back of the eye and even damage to the retina that doctors can see with a special light (an ophthalmoscope) shone into the eyes. In very severe cases of hypertension the nerve at the back of the eye may swell - this is an emergency. Sometimes a retinal vein or artery may be blocked, and this can cause partial or even total blindness in the affected eye.

Malignant Hypertension

I must also mention a condition known as malignant hypertension. 'Malignant' is a word usually used to describe some cancerous tumours, and malignant hypertension is every bit as awful as a malignant tumour. Often the blood pressure is extraordinarily high, with bleeding and fluid deposits in the retinas in the eyes and possible swelling of the optic nerves. There may be rapid deterioration in kidney function as well. Fortunately malignant hypertension is rare, but if it develops it must be treated urgently. Malignant hypertension tends not to creep up on patients but to occur suddenly for reasons that are not entirely clear. It requires hospital treatment and the administration of drugs that lower blood pressure very rapidly. Fortunately the survival of people with this rare condition is now much better with aggressive blood pressure-lowering treatment.

You may have found this chapter heavy going and may now feel like reaching for the anti-depressants. The remedy is simple: You have a much better chance of avoiding becoming a statistic or a vascular catastrophe by having your blood pressure taken and treated appropriately. Only by understanding the dangers of not treating hypertension can you cope successfully with it. The message is a positive one and there is no reason why anybody should put themselves at risk from any of these lethal but largely avoidable complications.

Chapter Six

Tests and Investigations

Once high blood pressure has come to light - though most people with hypertension have no symptoms unless there is also organ damage - your doctor, whether it be a GP or a hospital consultant, will carry out some routine tests, and possibly some more sophisticated investigations as well.

Medical History and Physical Examination

Your doctor will almost certainly ask you some detailed questions about your current and past medical history. For example, you will be questioned about chest pain, breathlessness or palpitations, as well as being asked direct questions about headaches and nose bleeds. Women will be questioned about whether they have had high blood pressure during pregnancy. The doctor may ask if there is any past history of kidney trouble - symptoms of this include passing overly large amounts of urine or passing urine at night. You will also be asked about smoking habits, alcohol and salt intake. The doctor will also want to know if there is any hypertension or diabetes in your family.

The physical exam may often reveal nothing apart from the presence of high blood pressure. The doctor will however, want to know how fast your pulse is beating, because a particularly fast pulse may indicate anxiety and this, in turn, may reflect on the measurement of blood pressure in the surgery. A fast pulse can sometimes be a sign of other conditions such as an overactive thyroid, while a slow pulse may indicate an underactive thyroid. Certain drugs such as beta-blockers can also slow the pulse.

The doctor may listen with a stethoscope over the arteries in your neck; if these arteries become narrowed they sometimes make a noise (a *bruit*). The doctor will listen to your heart to see if the intensity of the sounds is normal, as often in long-standing cases of high blood pressure one of the sounds is abnormally loud. There may also be additional heart sounds that suggest the heart is under some strain. The pulses in the wrists and in the groin should be felt simultaneously, because in coarctation of the aorta (see page 26), the pulses in the groin may be delayed. The purpose of listening to the chest is to make sure there are no signs of congestion of the lungs and to hear if there are any signs of obstruction to the airways. This is very important when it comes to deciding what medications can or cannot be given. The pulses in the feet should be checked to ensure there is no evidence of obstruction to the circulation to the legs. The eyes should also be examined (see Chapter Five).

Urine Sample

In the GP's surgery, or at a first visit to the hospital out-patients' department, a newly diagnosed hypertensive person should be asked to provide a sample of urine. There are little sticks that can be dipped into the specimen of urine which tell doctors whether there is any protein, sugar or blood in the urine. Protein and blood might suggest either a kidney abnormality as the cause of the high blood pressure, or kidney damage secondary to high blood pressure. Sugar in the urine can indicate that the person might have diabetes.

Blood Tests

If the person has not had a set of simple blood tests, then these should be organised by the doctor. Sometimes the blood tests are done as part of the Well Man/Woman screening mentioned previously. More often than not routine tests of the blood count, kidney and liver function will not reveal anything untoward. Nevertheless, there are certain abnormalities which can occur and which are certainly relevant to the patient with high blood pressure. For example, some people have too many red blood cells and an elevated haemoglobin level. This may suggest a condition called *polycythaemia* (which means 'too many cells'); there is an association between this and hypertension. The presence of anaemia might suggest an underlying kidney problem, while, in people who drink too much alcohol, the red blood cells actually become bigger - this can also be seen on the blood film.

Tests of kidney function are very important. If the kidneys are not working properly, then waste products called urea and creatinine accumulate in the blood. Measurements of the chemicals sodium, potassium and calcium in the blood may also give a clue as to any potential underlying cause of high blood pressure - although, as we will see in Chapters Seven and Eight, medications such as diuretics (commonly known as water pills) can alter the levels of these chemicals in the blood.

There really is no excuse for failing to run a simple set of blood biochemistry tests, because nearly all laboratories can measure a whole range of common chemicals, including cholesterol, uric acid (the chemical that causes gout) and tests of the kidneys, liver and thyroid all from a small volume of blood. There is, therefore, even less excuse for the medical profession to overlook any abnormal biochemical results.

ECG and X-ray

Some doctors will ask for an electrocardiogram (ECG) and a chest x-ray. Certain abnormalities might show up on the ECG. For example, if the heart muscle becomes excessively thickened, then the 'spikes' of each heartbeat shown on the ECG may be enlarged. If the heart muscle comes under a great deal of strain, then one of the wiggly lines (called a T-wave) which is normally upright on an ECG may be upside-down or inverted. Abnormal rhythms such as atrial fibrillation can also be detected.

The ECG is a very widely available test. It should be mentioned that, although there are certain well-defined limits of normality, factors other than disease can affect the appearance of the ECG. Although doctors commonly add up the size of the waves in parts of the ECG to help decide if the heart muscle is thickened or not, a very tall, thin patient may produce tall waves even if the heart muscle is not thick. Similarly, an overweight patient - with more bulk between his or her heart and the ECG machine - may well have a thickened heart muscle that nevertheless does not show up on the ECG. Some people just have 'a funny-looking ECG' even when there is absolutely nothing wrong with them. If a doctor is unsure as to whether a person's heart muscle is thickened or not, then an echocardiogram, also known as a cardiac ultrasound, may help.

A chest x-ray is not very helpful most of the time, unless the person has symptoms such as breathlessness. If the person is breathless, then a chest x-ray can tell doctors if the lungs are congested or if the heart is enlarged. If the lungs have been damaged by cigarette smoke, they will appear too dark. In people with a thickened heart muscle, the chest x-ray may still appear normal. For the vast majority of people with high blood pressure, the chest x-ray is probably the one test that could quite easily be dispensed with.

It is unlikely that your GP will request any more complicated tests than these. If your urine test is normal, if tests on the blood count, liver, kidney, thyroid and cholesterol are all normal, and if the ECG is normal, then the doctor has to make a decision about whether further tests are worthwhile. With people who give a family history of high blood pressure, further, more sophisticated tests are unlikely to prove very useful. If we follow the axiom that 'common things commonly occur', then it is perfectly reasonable in cases such as this for a doctor to abandon investigations at this stage and just start treatment. There is really very little point in putting a 55-year-old newly diagnosed hypertensive man through a whole series of complicated scans and urine collections if he tells you that both his parents, two uncles and two or three of his siblings have also got high blood pressure.

More Sophisticated Investigations

The 'doctor's dilemma' is to decide who merits more sophisticated tests. Some of these tests are very expensive and time-consuming, and not a little inconvenient to the patient. Part of the art of medicine is being able to make difficult clinical judgements. Sometimes young doctors, particularly in hospital, display enormous zeal to investigate everybody; senior doctors have to temper this enthusiasm with the hand of experience.

Professors Beevers and MacGregor have suggested nine criteria to ascertain whether a patient should undergo more sophisticated tests. These are:

1. If the doctor suspects an underlying secondary cause of the high

blood pressure, for example if there is any indication of one of the hormonal abnormalities mentioned previously, or if there is a discrepancy between the pulses in the wrist and the groin, or if the patient complains of episodes of severe flushing and palpitations.

2. 'Severe' hypertension. In the real world doctors will never agree on what constitutes severe (as opposed to moderate) hypertension. Most doctors would regard a systolic reading of 200mm/Hg or higher, and a diastolic of 110mm/Hg or higher, as severe, but in our far-from-ideal world not everyone with readings like this will receive sophisticated further investigations.

3. The young hypertensive person ('young' being anything more than 10 years younger than the doctor!) should probably have further investigations even if they have a family history of high blood pressure. Many younger hypertensives tell their doctor that their parents or grandparents had high blood pressure diagnosed in their sixties and seventies. Doctors may therefore feel that the person in front of them is a bit too young to be safely labelled as having essential or inherited high blood pressure. Let us remember, however, that just because your parents had hypertension diagnosed in later life does not mean that they did not have it for much longer, and of course previous generations had less access to health-screening and Well-person clinics than today's younger patients. How far a doctor investigates the younger patient will be a matter of individual clinical judgement.

4. If urine tests reveal protein, blood or glucose on dip-stick testing, then further tests should be carried out.

5. People with abnormal kidney biochemistry will need further tests.

6. People with a low potassium level in their blood (if they are not taking water pills) need investigation.

7. People who have been treated and who have failed to respond properly to medication should be further investigated.

8. People with large swings in blood pressure should be tested further, particularly if these swings are associated with other symptoms such as flushing and palpitations.

9. People who show a large drop in blood pressure when they move from being seated or lying down to a standing position should be

further investigated. Some of these may have deficiencies in the way blood pressure is regulated, and many may turn out to have diabetes.

So what are the further tests that the hypertensive person may have to go through?

Three of the most common are a) an ultrasound examination of the heart, b) a 24-hour urine collection, and c) an ultrasound examination of the kidneys.

Ultrasound Examination of the Heart

An ultrasound of the heart is a more accurate way than an ECG of measuring the thickness of the heart muscle. It can also show how the heart is contracting and relaxing, and give the doctor a look at the size of the upper chambers in people who have atrial fibrillation. Doctors can also look at the diameter of the aorta - the main blood vessel that comes out of the heart - to make sure it is not too dilated. Because this test is incredibly safe and easily repeatable, it can be used to follow how the heart is responding while blood pressure is being treated: with the proper treatment, a dilated heart may become smaller, and a thickened heart muscle can also return to normal.

24-hour Urine Collection

Several things can be measured from a 24-hour urine specimen. If simple blood tests indicate that the blood urea and creatinine levels are elevated, then the doctor may order a test known as a *creatinine clearance*. Kidney specialists who see a lot of hypertensive patients can use this to monitor how the kidneys are performing.

Protein measurements in the urine can also be made. Normally the kidneys do not leak protein out into the urine, but such a leak can be quantified and its progression or regression monitored. In people with diabetes, careful monitoring of protein in the urine is extremely important because, in this case, when protein appears in the urine it can predict the onset of kidney failure. Some of the more modern drugs can reduce the rate at which the kidneys leak protein (see Chapter Seven).

In people where the rare condition of phaeochromocytoma is suspected, a 24-hour urine sample can be used to measure the breakdown products of adrenaline and noradrenaline and related chemicals.

A 24-hour urine collection can be something of a burden. My recommendation is that the patient tries to do this over a weekend, perhaps starting on a Sunday morning and finishing on Monday morning so that, if possible, the bottle or container can be delivered back to the laboratory first thing Monday morning. It is absolutely imperative that urine be collected for the whole 24-hour period; many laboratories will now provide a large enough container in a fairly anonymous carrier bag to protect the sensitivities of fellow-passengers on buses and trains!

We should never underestimate the capacity of any laboratory to make mistakes, and it is important to stress to people doing a 24-hour urine collection for breakdown products of adrenaline that the bottle must be acidified. It really is very depressing to have done a meticulous 24-hour urine collection, only for the doctor to receive a rather pathetic apology from the laboratory that the container was wrong and it has to be done all over again.

Ultrasound Examination of the Kidneys

In the same way that the heart can be examined by ultrasound, so can the kidneys and most other structures in the abdomen. A renal ultrasound is particularly useful for looking at the size of the kidneys, checking if they are symmetrical or not, and looking for cysts or for any obstruction to the small tubes (ureters) that carry urine from each kidney to the bladder. The ultrasound scan can also pick up abnormalities in the adrenal glands on top of the kidneys and - one of the most overlooked uses for the ultrasound in clinical practice - can measure the diameter of the abdominal aorta. As mentioned in Chapter Five, in some cases of high blood pressure the abdominal aorta can swell silently with the passage of time, producing an aneurysm that may produce no symptoms until it starts to leak or it bursts.

In modern cardiac and renal ultrasound, 'flow' measurements can be made using the Doppler technique. The Doppler technique looks at the velocity of blood using a complex mathematical equation related to the change in wavelength of the ultrasound. At its simplest, we come across the Doppler effect most days of our lives when we hear a police car, ambulance or fire engine going past and the sound seems to change as the vehicle goes further away from us (that is, the wavelength of the sound changes). The reason I include this is that some radiologists will put in their reports, based on ultrasound exam alone, that the flow in the renal arteries is normal and, therefore, they believe they can exclude the condition of renal artery stenosis. Other radiologists are more careful, however, because the renal arteries can be very difficult to image in this way, as they are a long way from the ultrasound probe. Most doctors, therefore, would not accept an ultrasound scan as the best test for excluding this condition.

There are other tests that have more accuracy for detecting narrowing of the renal arteries, including a radioactive scan to see if the kidneys excrete symmetrically, although latterly this test has fallen into disfavour. The wide availability of CT scanning and magnetic resonance imaging (MRI) enables doctors to look at the kidneys, the adrenal glands and the renal arteries. MRI is particularly environmentally friendly as it does not use x-rays.

If a doctor really suspects a problem with the renal arteries, then a selective injection of iodine-containing contrast medium into the renal arteries can be carried out by a radiologist. This test is called a *renal angiogram*. Localised narrowings of the renal arteries can be treated at the same sitting by ballooning of the narrowed vessels to make them wider; this procedure is called *angioplasty*. A metal coil (stent) can also be placed in the artery to hold it open, in a technique which has evolved from the use of this treatment in coronary artery disease.

Other Tests

If your doctor thinks you have symptoms or signs of arterial disease affecting the heart or the brain, then a whole series of other tests up to and including angiograms of the coronary or carotid arteries may be ordered, but these are beyond the scope of this book.

24-hour Blood-pressure Monitor

The 24-hour ambulatory blood-pressure monitor (see page 34) method of assessing the blood pressure away from the stress and anxiety of hospital or a doctor's consulting room has proved very useful, especially so in those patients whose blood pressure measurements seem to fluctuate. It is a real dilemma for doctors treating hypertension to be presented with a little notebook of readings taken at home which are normal, and yet a separate list of readings that are abnormal which were taken by a hospital doctor or at the GP's surgery. The 'white coat syndrome' I referred to earlier is, in truth, probably overdiagnosed, but it is certainly true that there is a group of people who seem to have elevated blood pressures in a clinical environment even when they do not look stressed. A 24-hour blood pressure monitor may be particularly useful in people with borderline elevations of blood pressure who really do not want to be burdened with tablets for the rest of their lives. It is also true that a series of measurements over a 24-hour period provides a 'big picture' which can guide a doctor as to whether to give advice on lifestyle changes or to start prescribing medication.

It would be a big mistake, however, to dismiss patients who have high blood pressure when their doctors take it and yet a normal blood pressure when they monitor it themselves at home as 'normal'. Some of these people will go on to become true hypertensives with time.

The monitor is useful, too, for convincing people who do not believe they have high blood pressure, as they have only to see the readings they've obtained at home or at work and they will be left in no doubt.

Needless to say, the blood pressure monitor can also be used to follow the success or otherwise of treatment and also to ensure that treatment provides the round-the-clock protection which we now know to be incredibly important in saving lives.

A Word of Advice

Before we move on, a word of advice. Do not be alarmed if your doctor does not put you through all the battery of tests that I have described in this chapter. Most people do not have intrinsic kidney disease or esoteric adrenaline-producing tumours. Most people with high blood pressure just have it for genetic and biochemical reasons. People should never be disappointed if they are not 'an interesting case'. It is better to have something boring and common that doctors know how to treat, rather than something rare and interesting that leaves doctors perplexed and scratching their heads.

Chapter Seven

Treating High Blood Pressure

The next two chapters will make up the largest chunk of this book. Many people will have come across the phrase 'evidence-based medicine' in the newspapers. This has become a catchphrase in the medical profession and was born out of the finding that standards of medical care vary unacceptably in different parts of the country. Some GPs and hospital doctors were prescribing the latest fad treatments based on only scanty evidence of their effectiveness. At the other extreme, some doctors were failing to give their patients the benefit of newer treatments that had been subjected to rigorous medical testing and whose benefits had been proven beyond reasonable doubt.

Fortunately with hypertension there have been a large number of clinical trials conducted over many years. By re-examining medical research, it has become apparent that for each reduction of 10mm-14mm/Hg in systolic pressure and 5mm-6mm/Hg in diastolic blood pressure, the risk of stroke is lowered by about 40 per cent and the risk of coronary heart disease by about 15 per cent.

The Rule of Halves

The rule of halves described in Chapter Four is not confined to the United Kingdom. International studies of clinical practice have provided a devastating indictment of the inadequate treatment of hypertension. In 1999 a paper was published in a *European Heart Journal* supplement. The percentages of hypertensive patients with blood pressures controlled to 140/90 or better in different countries were shown. The United States topped the list, with 27.4 per cent of hypertensives having adequate control, Germany had 22.5 per cent, Finland 20.5 per cent, Spain 20 per cent, Australia 19 per cent, Scotland 17.5 per cent, Canada 16 per cent, India 9 per cent, and England 5.9 per cent - beaten to bottom spot in this survey only by Zaire, with 2.5. The Americans should not be particularly proud of their 27.4 per cent, but in England the level of blood pressure control can only be described as lamentable.

There are several possible reasons for this poor performance.

- Overworked general practitioners may fail to monitor patients' blood pressure on medication.
- Patients may believe that once their initial prescription runs out they do not need to renew it.
- Patients may not feel like continuing on medication because they have no symptoms to start with.
- A drug may have side-effects which some patients may find unacceptable and, therefore, discontinue the drug on their own.
- Other patients might wish to report the side-effects to their general practitioner but find they cannot get an appointment and, therefore, just abandon the pills.

Reasons are not excuses, however, and it is up to health professionals to digest the best clinical trials and prescribe the right drugs to the right patients.

There are far too many clinical trials on high blood pressure to mention in this book, although individual reference will be made to some of the modern ones where they are relevant.

What the studies have taught us is that blood pressure must not be seen in isolation. In 1998 a study from Gothenburg was published in the *British Medical Journal*. This study, which began in 1970, compared the survival over a 20-year period of 686 hypertensive men between the ages of 47 and 55 years, with the survival of a control group (i.e. patients of similar ages, lifestyles and smoking habits) of 6,810 people with normal blood pressure. In spite of achieving good blood pressure control, and in spite of lowering cholesterol and reducing cigarette smoking from 34 per cent to 17 per cent, the hypertensive group still had a worse survival rate than the other group, with deaths from heart attacks predominating. After 20 years there was just under an 80 per cent chance that the patients with normal blood pressure would be alive, and only about a 70 per cent chance that the treated hypertensive people would be alive.

Although any piece of published research has flaws and criticisms which can be applied to it (there were more smokers and worse cholesterol levels in the hypertensive group than in the control group), the finding in this Swedish study did not come as a total surprise. This study, like many other earlier studies, may have been a bit too lax in the blood pressure targets. We now like to have a much tighter control of blood pressure.

Global Risk

Equally important is the recognition of global risk. In Chapter Two I referred to the relevance of obesity, lack of exercise and excess salt along with other factors such as cigarette smoking, an abnormal cholesterol profile and diabetes. Some doctors with a special interest in high blood pressure recommend that every GP or hospital doctor who is responsible for hypertensive patients should use a risk-profiling chart or a computer programme. If the chart or programme indicates that any patient has a 15 per cent chance or greater of developing heart disease over the next 10 years, then treatment should be started.

I tend to disagree with the 'medicine by numbers' approach to treatment. What about the patients with a 12 or 13 per cent risk? Are they not to be treated, too? Those who challenge my question will probably say that doctors should use their common sense - and that is exactly my point! I prefer a clinical common-sense approach to the treatment of hypertension, in the same way that I would hope to adopt a sensible approach to treating a high cholesterol or on advising a patient whether to take aspirin or not.

The concept of global risk really allows us to rephrase 'treatment of hypertension' as 'management of hypertension'. So, before condemning people to a lifetime of drug treatment, it is worth examining some of the lifestyle alterations that might lower blood pressure. Although none of the trials has shown conclusively that reducing blood pressure through lifestyle changes actually prevents heart attacks or strokes, it is quite logical for doctors to advise on lifestyle issues given that the reduction of blood pressure by any means reduces the risks of heart attacks and strokes.

In October 2000, Dr Jonathan Morrell, a general practitioner in Surrey, published a paper in a journal called *Modern Hypertension*

Management in which he reviewed the benefits of lifestyle changes on blood pressure, having studied a large number of clinical trials. The results can be summarised as follows:

1. A 3-9 per cent loss in body weight will reduce systolic and diastolic blood pressure by 3mm/Hg.
2. A low-fat, high fruit and vegetable diet will reduce systolic blood pressure by 5.5mm/Hg and diastolic blood pressure by 3mm/Hg.
3. Fifteen minutes of aerobic exercise three times a week will reduce systolic blood pressure by 5mm/Hg and diastolic blood pressure by 3mm/Hg.
4. Salt restriction reduces systolic blood pressure by 4mm/Hg and diastolic blood pressure by 2mm/Hg. Potassium supplementation will reduce systolic blood pressure by 4.4mm/Hg and diastolic blood pressure by 2.5mm/Hg (this may be one of the reasons why a high fruit and vegetable intake are beneficial, as potassium is found in these foods). There is no role for potassium tablets in lowering blood pressure.
5. Fish oil supplementation of up to 3g per day reduces systolic blood pressure by 4.5mm/Hg and diastolic blood pressure by 2.5mm/Hg.

These reductions may sound small, but they may make the difference between having to take tablets or not. So an overweight patient who manages to lose weight, restrict salt intake and take some exercise may escape the monthly visit to the local pharmacist!

The major drawback of all these lifestyle research studies is that they were of short duration. However, looking on the bright side, even if these modifications postpone the need for taking tablets for five years or so, that is hardly a bad thing for the individual patient - or for the national drug bill.

Hawk-eyed readers will have noticed that stopping smoking does not appear in the above list. It is worth reiterating that quitting smoking is probably the single most effective lifestyle modification that any smoker can make, but its benefits are probably not related to an effect on blood pressure. Given that smoking compounds the risk to hypertensive people of developing furred-up and blocked arteries, it is desperately important that anybody with high blood pressure stops smoking.

We have referred to stress in ChapterTwo and, of course, it is difficult to quantify stress and draw a graph relating stress to high blood pressure. Most doctors, however, will be able to recall patients with hypertension who were particularly bad at managing their time. These people spend their whole lives chasing deadlines and targets or dashing from one meeting to another, or pass hours sitting in an aircraft seat or at business lunches. This sort of lifestyle is not necessarily conducive to a careful assessment of diet and salt intake, nor will it leave much time for exercise. Stress-management should, therefore, include attention to other details. I have known people who have managed to find another job within the same organisation and their blood pressure has fallen to normal. There is no reason why a hypertensive person in any job cannot at least make some effort to lower blood pressure with lifestyle management. A long-distance lorry driver who eats junk food, drinks 10 pints of beer a day, smokes like a chimney and takes no exercise has just as good a chance of reducing his coronary risk as the high-flying executive who has two business meals a day with excess salt and who laments the lack of time for exercise. The common factor in both these cases is the desire to change the way they live and perhaps to manage their time better. It is the same for smoking. Those who really want to stop find it easier to do so than those who do not!

My own family will scarcely be able to contain their mirth at these lofty sentiments. Here is a doctor with a busy NHS and private medical practice, who rarely gets home before 9.30 at night and who can never have a meal or a game of tennis without being interrupted by the shrill tones of a pager or a mobile phone! However, at least my interrupted meals are healthy ones and, come rain or shine, I do make the effort to get to the tennis court. The facts of life are that it may not be possible for anybody in a challenging job with long hours and lots of stress to abandon this job for a beach hut in the Seychelles, but some changes are usually possible when necessary.

Another way of stress reduction is meditation. Transcendental meditation can be very effective, even for sceptics. A study published in the journal *Hypertension* in 1995 reported that in 127 African-Americans aged between 55 and 85 years, TM was twice as effective as other techniques such as progressive muscle relaxation, and produced an average of nearly 11mm/Hg reduction in systolic pressure compared with people who did not meditate.

Prescribing Anti-hypertensive Medication

Those people who are facing anti-hypertensive medication now do not realise how lucky they are compared to their counterparts of 30 years ago. The first anti-hypertensive drugs were introduced in the 1950s, but they had such bad side-effects that they were only used in people with malignant hypertension or with terrible symptoms. Before these drugs came in, people with hypertension were placed on total bed-rest and given sedatives or tranquillisers. Some people even had operations to cut the sympathetic nerves or to have their adrenal glands removed. In the late 1960s and early 1970s beta-blockers and diuretics (water pills) became available, but before these came on to the market, the main blood pressure-lowering drugs were the group known as the adrenergic neurone-blockers - but patients hated them. They made people dizzy when they stood up and they caused impotence in men. This explains why blood pressure pills were so unpopular. Why on earth should anybody take a medication that makes them feel worse than they did before, given that the condition that is being treated usually has no symptoms?

Although modern drugs are much better and there is a huge variety, it is sometimes still difficult to persuade people to take a pill, especially when they are young, active and possess that sense of immortality which we all have at a certain age. There is often a natural resentment felt by newly diagnosed hypertensive people that they are condemned to a life of taking tablets. Few of us, other than the most entrenched hypochondriacs, actually enjoy taking pills. Doctors have a duty to make patients see beyond the 'Why me?' syndrome. My own approach in this situation is to ask patients how they would feel if they were told that they had diabetes, which may also be picked up on routine testing and also produce no symptoms. People with diabetes may accept the need for tablets or even for insulin injections without demurring. Perhaps this is because most people know that diabetes is a serious condition which can cause terrible complications in later life, but maybe we have failed to educate the public that hypertension is no less dangerous a condition.

There are a few general principles with which most doctors would agree for prescribing medication to control hypertension:

1. Doctors should not use a drug that can be predicted to cause a side-effect. The most common example here is the use of beta-blocking drugs in patients who have asthma.
2. It is preferable to use a long-acting drug that provides 24-hour control and needs to be taken only once a day. This type of 24-hour control protects against the surges of blood pressure in the morning hours that are associated with the greatest chance of sudden death, heart attacks and strokes (described in Chapter Five). In addition, people are less likely to forget a once-a-day drug than one that needs to be taken three times a day.
3. Doctors should start patients on a low dose. A small dose of a drug can always be increased, but if the dose is too big and the patients develop side-effects, then they may lose confidence in that medication and be reluctant to continue with it.
4. A small dose of a second or even a third drug can be added over a period of time. It is much better for a patient to take three tablets and have no side-effects than to take one tablet at so high a dose that, while it may well work, it causes unacceptable side-effects.
5. Doctors must not panic if the patient's blood pressure does not come under control immediately. It may take up to six weeks for a drug to produce its maximum effect, and the worst thing doctors can do is to keep chopping and changing medication without giving each one a reasonable amount of time to work. Only in the most severe cases of hypertension or malignant hypertension is a very rapid reduction in blood pressure necessary.
6. If patients truly do not respond to a drug or have terrible side-effects, then they should be changed to another class of drugs.

In spite of all the biochemical and hormonal research which has improved our understanding of hypertension, there is very little rocket science when it comes to prescribing a medication for an individual patient. In an ideal world, doctors would assess each patient and decide which particular drug was best for him or her. It has been suggested that doctors should ask themselves what anti-hypertensive *they* would take if they themselves needed some medication - this often helps to concentrate the mind! Sometimes it can be quite simple to customise treatment. For example, a very anxious person with a persistently high pulse rate and high blood pressure may have a good response to a beta-blocker. These are the exception rather than the rule, although in most cases it does not matter what we use as long as the end result is a controlled blood pressure.

Anti-hypertensive Drugs

There are six main classes of anti-hypertensives available, and three or four subsidiary classes which are used less commonly. You will hopefully understand that I neither can nor should attempt to explain the benefits and drawbacks of every single anti-hypertensive drug that is available on prescription - I would need far too much space! I will instead cover the classes of drug in general terms, and describe some of the benefits and side-effects that each class of drug may produce.

The six main classes of drugs are:
1. Diuretics
2. Beta-blockers
3. Calcium channel-blockers
4. ACE-inhibitors
5. Angiotensin II receptor-blockers
6. Alpha-blockers

Do not worry if *alpha* and *beta* are all Greek to you at the moment, as all will be revealed shortly!

Diuretics
Diuretics are commonly known as water pills and they are prescribed to millions of people around the world to help them get rid of excess fluid. The most common cause of the excess fluid is heart failure. There are many diuretics on the market, some weak and some strong, which clear fluid from congested lungs and tissues and which make patients with heart failure feel very much better.

All diuretics make people urinate frequently. They act on the kidneys to make them pump out salt and water from the body - anyone who has taken a diuretic will know that the frequent trips to the toilet can sometimes play havoc with your working and social life.

One group of diuretics is particularly useful for hypertension. These drugs, known as thiazides, often have long names usually ending in '-iazide'. Sometimes diuretics are given inappropriately by doctors, possibly to people who feel they want to lose some weight. These people may become extremely dizzy as their blood pressure drops precipitously. When given appropriately to hypertensives, diuretics may produce adequate control on their own, and many people have been taking these drugs for a long time with no untoward effects. Sometimes diuretics are given in combination with other medications.

People who are given thiazides for hypertension may notice that they pass large quantities of urine for a few days, but even when this particular phenomenon tails off the blood pressure-lowering effect may be maintained. There is some evidence that in addition to helping the body lose salt and water, thiazides may dilate arteries directly and hence lower blood pressure by another action.

Serious side-effects are rare with thiazides. A very small number of people develop skin rashes and abnormalities of the white blood cells or platelet cells, but the most inconvenient side-effect is sexual impotence in males. We will come back to erectile dysfunction later on, but although it is worth sexually active males trying thiazides, it is impossible to persuade people to persevere with thiazide if it spoils their sex life.

Other thiazide side-effects are related to blood chemistry. As these drugs make your body lose salt and water, they can also cause loss of potassium. A low potassium may have no deleterious effect in people whose heart function is normal, but in people with damaged hearts, such as those who have suffered heart attacks or whose heart muscle has been damaged by long-term hypertension, low potassium levels can put you at risk of quite serious rhythm disturbances. Your doctor needs to be on the ball here and make sure that your potassium levels are measured regularly. Some of the thiazide diuretics come with built-in potassium supplements to counteract this - these drugs usually end with a capital K (K being the symbol for potassium). Some people can lose quite dramatic amounts of potassium which will not be adequately replaced by the small supplement in the pill, so even if you are taking one of these preparations you must have your potassium levels checked regularly. Sometimes specific potassium supplements can be given although these are often unpleasant, even in the fizzy form. Another option is to eat foods high in potassium such as tomatoes and bananas.

Some of the other anti-hypertensives actually help the body conserve potassium, so when these are used in conjunction with thiazides, potassium loss is less of a problem.

Another occasional side-effect of thiazides is a rise in the blood sugar level. Nearly always this is just a biochemical reaction with little clinical importance, but in some cases the blood sugar level may rise quite markedly. Even more rarely, people may develop full-blown diabetes. Doctors try to avoid prescribing thiazide diuretics for people with diabetes, although if they are thought to be absolutely necessary, the dose of insulin or sugar-lowering drugs might need to be adjusted.

Gout may occur if the uric acid in the blood becomes elevated. Thiazides may increase the levels of uric acid in the blood, but unless this precipitates an attack of gout or is associated with kidney stones, you should not worry too much about it. In people who have a tendency to gout, doctors will try to avoid prescribing thiazides if at all possible.

Less important biochemical alterations associated with thiazides include an occasional rise in cholesterol and calcium levels in the blood. You might think that a blood pressure pill which elevates blood cholesterol would be undoing some of the benefits that are achieved by lowering blood pressure. However this is not the case; the overall benefits of lowering blood pressure vastly outweigh the small rise in blood cholesterol. Markedly raised calcium levels are rarely a problem in clinical practice, but if they do occur then they may prompt further investigation of your parathyroid glands, which are close to the thyroid gland in the neck.

There are also one or two other non-thiazide diuretics that your doctor may want to give you, some of which may help conserve potassium.

Beta-blockers

In Chapter Three I wrote that the sympathetic nervous system is part of what we call the autonomic nervous system, out of our voluntary control. The sympathetic nervous system controls our response to physical or emotional stress and helps with the 'flight or fight reaction'. Sympathetic reaction is brought about by adrenaline and related compounds. For many years doctors have divided the sympathetic nervous system into two classes, according to the receptors in the organs that the sympathetic nervous system is controlling. These are described as alpha receptors and beta receptors. The beta receptors are further divided into beta 1 and beta 2. Don't worry, it doesn't get much more complicated!

A *receptor* is an area on a blood vessel or an organ to which a chemical attaches itself in order to exert its influence on that blood vessel or organ. A receptor-blocker simply attaches itself to the receptor site like a barnacle on a rock and prevents the active chemical from having its way. Receptor-blockers have to compete with the chemical for the receptor site in the same way that two children may compete for one chair in a game of musical chairs! Beta 1 receptors control the rate at which the heart beats and how powerfully it contracts. Beta 2 receptors make blood vessels dilate, but may narrow the airways in the lungs. This can be a big problem in people with asthma or other forms of chronic lung disease. Beta-blockers also reduce renin release from the kidneys, so there is less angiotensin II around (which reduces constriction of the arteries).

The alpha-blockers are our sixth class of anti-hypertensive, and alpha actions, which are generally less important than beta actions are discussed on page 83.

Beta-blockers have several potential ways of lowering blood pressure. If the heart rate and the force of contraction of the heart are reduced, if arteries in muscles dilate and the constricting effect of angiotensin II is diminished, then blood pressure should fall. Beta-blockers are also used to treat angina sufferers, because reducing the heart rate and the force of contraction reduces the amount of oxygen the heart needs, and so helps alleviate angina.

It is very doubtful whether slowing the heart down and reducing its force of contraction contributes much to the lowering of blood pressure in hypertensive people. It is probably beta-blockers' action in reducing renin levels that is their most powerful role in managing hypertension.

Several beta-blockers have come and gone since they were first introduced in the 1960s, but there are still a large number on the market. Beta-blockers nearly always end in '-olol'. The manufacturers will have trade names for them, as with any drug, but it is helpful if patients know the generic rather than brand name of the drug they are taking. Although one doctor may prescribe a particular brand and use its trade name, another doctor, particularly in another country, may not be so familiar with that drug. The generic (or true) names are the same around the world.

The manufacturers of beta-blockers have spent an enormous amount of time and money marketing their individual products and trying to persuade both GPs and hospital doctors that their own beta-blocker is better than that of their competitors'. Opinion is divided in the medical profession as to whether one beta-blocker is actually better than another, although there are some newer ones that have become available in the last few years that may have fewer side-effects.

One of the major differences between them is that some beta-blockers are more active on the beta 1 receptors (that is, they have more effects on the heart). Others attack both beta 1 and beta 2 receptors equally. The ones that act only on beta 1 receptors are known as 'cardio-selective'. Theoretically, cardio-selective beta-blockers that do not constrict the airways in the lungs should be better tolerated by people with airways disease or asthma. Here things get a little bit tricky, because some people who do not have asthma may become quite wheezy on a beta-blocker but are quite all right when they are not taking one. Most doctors agree that all beta-blockers should be avoided in people with real asthma.

Some of the older beta-blockers had to be taken two or three times a day, which led to them being less effective simply because people forgot to take them. Some of these are now available in long-acting preparations. The newer beta-blockers do provide a full 24-hour action. Some even have a longer action and may take four or five days to get out of the system.

Until the mid 1980s beta-blockers and diuretics were the first-choice drugs for high blood pressure. The side-effects have made them less popular in more recent years. They remain of great benefit for people with angina and for those who have suffered a heart attack.

Not all beta-blockers cause all side-effects in all people. I have mentioned spasm of the airways, wheezing and asthma; other side-effects include a general feeling of lethargy and lack of mental alertness, inability to exercise properly, insomnia and nightmares. The blood vessels in the legs may constrict, which can cause cramp in the calves or buttocks, known as claudication. Excess slowing of the pulse rate can lead to dizziness and lethargy. Heart failure can occur if the force of contraction of the heart is reduced excessively. Last but not least, I'm afraid, is impotence.

The reason some beta-blockers can cause nightmares or sleep disturbances is that they are soluble in fats. A fat-soluble beta-blocker can cross the barrier between the blood and the brain. Sometimes these nightmares can be vivid and terrifying. If you are on a beta-blocker and it has no side-effects apart from nightmares, then your doctor should be able to find one that does not cross the blood-brain barrier, to give you a good night's sleep.

Beta-blockers are best avoided in people who have developed vascular disease in their legs. Even in people with fairly mild narrowings of their leg arteries, claudication can be produced - though it resolves rapidly once the beta-blocker is stopped. Some people complain bitterly about cold hands and cold feet even if they do not have any disease of their blood vessels, and this will necessitate stopping the beta-blocker.

In people with heart failure, beta-blockers must be used very cautiously. Until recently they were avoided because they could make heart failure worse. Medical thinking has altered recently and beta-blockers may be beneficial for some of these people, although they should only be given under strict medical supervision.

Beta-blockers are best avoided if you have a slow pulse already, or if there is evidence of problems with the electrical conduction pathways in the heart on an ECG.

Loss of energy, mental dullness and reduced exercise tolerance are less obvious side-effects than a severe wheeze or a pair of ice-cold hands. I am not alone in having grave doubts about the use of beta-blockers as first-line drugs, particularly in younger people with physically and mentally demanding jobs. As a medical student I participated in an experiment where I was given a beta-blocker and asked to cycle for 20 minutes. I felt I was pedalling uphill with 10-tonne weights attached to each leg - the experiment could not end quickly enough for me!

Doctors have traditionally been advised to avoid prescribing beta-blockers for people with insulin-dependent diabetes. Beta-blockers can disguise the symptoms of an excessively low blood sugar level (hypoglycaemia). If a patient's blood sugar level drops extremely low and the beta-blockers prevent the usual symptoms, the condition might not be recognised and this could prove dangerous or even fatal. However, in modern-day clinical practice and with better management and supervision of people with diabetes, there is no real reason why even those with insulin-dependent diabetes cannot be prescribed beta-blockers if necessary.

The Calcium Channel-blockers

These drugs have absolutely nothing to do with calcium in milk, bones or teeth, and so you are not about to find your bones collapsing or your teeth falling out if you are given one of these drugs! Calcium is very important in controlling the contraction and relaxation of the muscular coat of blood vessels; calcium-blockers work by reducing the amount of calcium that is available to these muscle cells and causing the arteries to relax and dilate.

Within the category of calcium channel-blockers are three major sub-groups. As two of the sub-groups at the time of writing this book only have one drug each in them, I am going to break my rule and mention them by name.

Dihydropyridines

The first group are called dihydropyridines. There are quite a few of these drugs available and their names end in '-ipine'. Some of them are long-acting and some short-acting, and some may be given when blood pressure needs to be lowered very quickly. Some of them are now available in once-a-day preparations which produce 24-hour control. These drugs are now widely used as first-line anti-hypertensives. They do not have any effects on blood biochemistry (including potassium and blood sugar). They may be used on their own or in combination with other drugs, and they do not upset the kidneys.

One of the most troublesome side-effects is swelling of the ankles. This is not because the drugs cause heart failure, but probably because they make capillaries leaky. Capillaries are the very small blood vessels which we cannot see in the tissues, and if water leaks out from them into the tissues, then those tissues can swell up. Due to the effects of gravity this is most commonly noticed in the legs, although some people will notice that their fingers feel swollen. Sometimes, particularly with the long-acting drugs, a reduction in the dose may help, but occasionally this symptom is really troublesome and the drug needs to be stopped. Many doctors mistakenly believe that giving a diuretic will get rid of the fluid from the tissues. Although this may help for a few people, it is usually of no benefit.

Another side-effect of these drugs can be a sensation of profound flushing, particularly in the face, possibly with a headache and a sensation of rapid palpitations. This side-effect is less common with the slow-release or long-acting preparations. This is caused by a rapid dilatation of the blood vessels, which makes the face feel flushed and, as a result of the rather abrupt lowering in blood pressure, the heart beats faster to try to keep the blood pressure up! Some people find the sensation of a rapid pulse rate very troublesome, but this side-effect can often be relieved by combining the drug with a beta-blocker.

More unusual side-effects include enlargement of the gums and, in middle-aged men, a need to get up and pass urine at night.

Verapamil

In the calcium channel-blocker group but completely different from the '-ipine' drugs is Verapamil. This is a much less powerful dilator of blood vessels but it has a more profound effect on the heart's rhythm. It was first used intravenously to treat rapid cardiac rhythm disorders, and is still used to prevent palpitations in some people while also finding a niche in the treatment of hypertension. The conventional preparation has to be given three times a day, but there are also long-acting preparations available.

Because it can slow the pulse, the general advice is that Verapamil should not be given with a beta-blocker, although there are a large number of patients taking Verapamil and a beta-blocker with no problem. Your doctor just has to be careful that there is no absolute reason not to use them together, to make sure he or she monitors your pulse rate regularly and to ask you specifically about any symptoms of an excessively slow pulse rate, such as dizziness or blackouts.

The other troublesome side-effect of Verapamil is constipation. This can be very severe in patients who tend to have constipation already. More often than not it can be overcome by the use of a high-fibre diet, which is what we should all be following anyway.

Diltiazem

The third drug in a group of its own is called Diltiazem, which is a very good drug for treating angina. It is commonly used in some countries as a first-line anti-hypertensive, although less widely in the United Kingdom. It can come in a variety of long-acting preparations which usually have the letters '-zem' somewhere in the name. Like Verapamil, it does not tend to cause flushing or palpitation but may cause troublesome ankle-swelling in some patients.

ACE-inhibitors

These drugs have made a huge difference to the management of cardiovascular disease. They block the conversion of angiotensin I to the powerful arteriolar-constrictor angiotensin II. They have been enormously successful in treating hypertension, both on their own or in combination with other drugs such as diuretics and calcium channel-blockers. They do not combine so effectively with beta-blockers.

The ACE-inhibitor drugs all end in '-pril'. As with beta-blockers 20 years ago, the market has exploded with many ACE-inhibitors and each manufacturer will claim that their ACE-inhibitor has subtle advantages over its competitors. In terms of blood pressure control, there are really no major differences between the ACE-inhibitors apart from whether they work for 24 hours or need to be taken three times a day.

One ACE-inhibitor in particular has been subjected to a very large and well-funded clinical trial whose results showed the drug to be of benefit to patients with coronary artery disease. This study attracted a great deal of media attention, as a result of which there was pressure on doctors to change patients from their existing ACE-inhibitor to this particular one, as the other ACE-inhibitors had not been shown to produce this benefit. What this means is that just because other ACE-inhibitors have not been subjected to the same clinical trials, it does not mean they haven't got a protective action on arteries as well. It is just that the trials have not been done on each individual drug.

Thickening of blood vessel walls and of the heart muscle can be produced by high levels of ACE in the tissues. There is increasing evidence that ACE-inhibitors can stop or even reverse this process.

These drugs have been shown to be very beneficial for people with heart failure of virtually any cause, independent of their blood pressure-lowering effect. They have been shown to prolong life in people with heart failure, and it is now almost mandatory for such patients, if at all possible, to be on one of these drugs in addition to diuretics and other medication.

Another recently discovered advantage of ACE-inhibitors is their beneficial effects on the kidneys for people with diabetes. They slow down the rate at which the diabetic kidneys lose protein, and delay the rate of onset of kidney failure. Nearly all diabetes specialists will have their patients on an ACE-inhibitor.

The most significant side-effect is a dry, irritating cough which can drive you and your relatives mad! It occurs in up to 15 to 20 per cent of patients. If you develop a cough on one ACE-inhibitor, you are likely to get the same cough if given another ACE-inhibitor instead. The cough can be particularly bad at night and, even if you do not have a cough due to the drug, a cough associated with a cold or flu may not clear until the ACE-inhibitor is stopped. Even then it may take six to eight weeks for the cough to completely clear. It is amazing how many patients put up with an ACE-inhibitor cough and how often neither they nor their doctors will make the association between the drug and the cough. The cough is caused by the build-up of a chemical called bradykinin as a side-effect of the drug's action.

Another side-effect of ACE-inhibitors, almost unique amongst anti-hypertensives, is an allergic reaction of swelling of the lips and the tongue and, fortunately more rarely, of obstruction of the airways. This condition is called angio-oedema. This condition is more common than many doctors have realised. If it arises, it signals a firm indication to stop the drug.

Sometimes ACE-inhibitors may interfere with kidney function, particularly if given with too big a dose of diuretics and particularly if there is renal artery stenosis (see Chapter Three). Some kidney specialists say that ACE-inhibitors can be used cautiously in people with this condition, but generally they are best avoided. If they are used, kidney function must be monitored regularly by blood tests. If a person given an ACE-inhibitor suddenly shows an unexpected deterioration in kidney function, then the doctor should suspect the presence of renal artery stenosis.

Another combination that can cause deterioration of kidney function is when ACE-inhibitors are used in conjunction with drugs that are used commonly for aches and pains in the joints. These are called non-steroidal anti-inflammatory drugs (NSAIDs). This can be a real problem because a) some doctors are not aware of this interaction, and b) sometimes people are taking these drugs without their doctor's knowledge. The good news is that when the drugs are stopped, the kidney function nearly always goes back to normal.

The ACE-inhibitors are widely prescribed as first-line anti-hypertensives and, unless people develop a cough, they are very well tolerated. They are also less likely to cause impotence than other drugs. They also help to conserve potassium, and so may offset the potassium loss the patient experiences with thiazide diuretics. They have revolutionised the treatment of hypertension.

Angiotensin II Receptor-antagonists

These are the next generation after the ACE-inhibitors. They generally provide a greater blockade of the action of angiotensin II. Instead of just preventing it from being manufactured, the receptor-antagonists act in the same way as beta-blockers do against adrenaline by preventing the angiotensin II from attaching itself to the arteries. These drugs are all known as '-sartans'. There are about five or six on the market at the time of writing this book, but a great many more are expected to come on the market. The better ones block the receptors completely and provide what some medical articles describe as an 'insurmountable blockade'.

Some of the '-sartans' are better than others; the newer ones are not only better at blocking the receptors but also have a good dose-response curve. This means that as you increase the dose, you get a bigger reduction in blood pressure. If you are on one of these, it is worth checking with your doctor that you are on one of the newer and more effective ones rather than the prototype.

The major advantage of these over the ACE-inhibitors is they hardly ever cause a cough. In fact, they are remarkably free of side-effects. Studies which have compared these drugs with placebos (tablets containing no active ingredient) have shown that people on a placebo had more side-effects than those on the '-sartans'! I cannot say that no patient will ever have a cough on one of these drugs, but it is extremely rare. In addition, they do not tend to cause angio-oedema, although some people may notice slight congestion of the nose as if they had got a cold, and very occasionally low back pain may occur.

Although they have not been around as long as the ACE-inhibitors, new research suggests that they may be just as beneficial as ACE-inhibitors in people with heart failure, although the jury is still out on this. They also seem to have the same protective action on the kidneys of patients with diabetes as the ACE-inhibitors. Many clinicians are now using these drugs as first-line anti-hypertensives, either alone or in combination with diuretics.

Alpha-blockers
The final main class of anti-hypertensive are the alpha-blockers, which lead to relaxation of arteries and veins and can lower cholesterol levels slightly, though we do not understand how. There are only one or two that are now used in everyday clinical practice and their names end in '-azocin'. They are not usually given as first-line drugs, but can be useful when added in to a cocktail of diuretics or beta-blockers if these latter two do not work adequately on their own or in combination. Because they dilate both arteries and veins, one of their side-effects is a drop in blood pressure upon standing up, a phenomenon known as *postural hypotension*.

One benefit of alpha-blockers is that they can relieve the symptoms of prostate trouble in middle-aged and elderly males. They do this by relaxing the neck of the bladder, making it easier to pass urine. Many urologists prescribe these drugs as an alternative to prostate surgery, which can only be a good thing!

Other Drugs

There are four or five other drugs around which do not actually conform to any of the aforementioned groups.

Labetalol
Labetalol is the only drug available which acts as both an alpha- and beta-blocker. Although this can be very useful in emergencies to lower blood pressure quickly, it does not have a great role in clinical practice nowadays. It may, however, be useful in pregnancy.

Two drugs that are rarely used nowadays act on alpha-receptors in the brain. These are known as Methyldopa and Clonidine respectively.

Methyldopa
Methyldopa was used a great deal in the 1960s and 1970s, but it often makes people feel very sleepy and depressed. It may also cause impotence. It is rarely used nowadays except in desperate circumstances when nothing else seems to work. It has, at least, been shown to be safe in pregnancy.

Clonidine
Clonidine had a problem, as although blood pressure initially responded quite well, it used to creep up again, necessitating the dose to be increased further and further. However, the main worry with it was that if a dose was omitted, blood pressure could shoot up to very high levels. This was a particular problem in patients taking Clonidine in addition to a beta-blocker. Now that there are so many other better and safer drugs around, Clonidine is hardly ever used.

Hydralazine
Hydralazine is a very powerful dilator of arteries and, again, is hardly ever used now, because of the rapid palpitations that it causes, along with symptoms of flushing, rather like those caused by the '-ipine' drugs. The drug can also occasionally induce quite a serious set of symptoms where patients suffer temperatures, joint pains, skin rashes and general malaise. For this reason it is hardly ever used in modern practice.

Moxonidine

My final drug is relatively new, and acts on receptors in the brain. This drug is called Moxonidine and has not yet found a role as a first-line anti-hypertensive but can be very useful as an add-on drug when three or four medications are needed. It does not cause fatigue or depression. The only side-effect I have come across in higher doses is a dry mouth.

So, I have taken you through the major classes of anti-hypertensives, how they work and what their main side-effects are. It is time to move on to a description of how doctors choose drugs in clinical practice and why you are likely to be given one drug as opposed to another, and what should happen once treatment has been started. You may be surprised by what you are about to read in Chapter Eight.

Chapter Eight

Treatment: What You Need to Know

In Chapter Seven I covered the six main classes of anti-hypertensives and how they work. There are so many different drugs available that if people on anti-hypertensive treatment get together and discuss their tablets, they will rarely find that they are taking identical drugs. It does not matter if patients are on a different drug or combination of drugs, except where there are firm indications to give specific drugs such as an ACE-inhibitor or an angiotensin receptor-blocker to patients with diabetes. People who have angina as well as hypertension may be better off on a beta-blocker or a calcium channel-blocker, which treat both problems.

The fact that there are so many different drugs available reflects the rather subjective nature of treating hypertension and the lack of perfect science. This differs completely from, for example, the treatment of severe infections where microbiologists would work very hard to culture the germ responsible and ensure that the prescribed antibiotic had the best chance of wiping out the infection.

What your doctor prescribes may come down to his or her own personal preference or experience, but there are also market forces at play. The pharmaceutical companies send representatives to both GPs and hospital doctors to try to persuade them that their drug is the best one and should be prescribed. These companies will often arrange for a consultant to give lectures at evenings or weekends to GPs to bring them up to date on the newer anti-hypertensives. I have done many of these presentations myself. It is important for credibility, however, that the lecturer does not push the drug manufactured by the company sponsoring the meeting too hard and make outrageous claims about its superiority over other drugs. The drug company representatives will usually be armed with the latest research data on their drugs; this is one of the ways that new information is distributed among the profession. Very few doctors would be persuaded to use a drug that is inferior to other medications simply because the drug company representatives supplied them with free samples, rubber tourniquets, or a few rather cheap ballpoint pens with the drug company's logo on them!

Economics are another factor in the choice of anti-hypertensives, as counterbalancing the sophisticated marketing campaigns of the drug industry are intense pressures to keep costs under control. In the UK primary care trusts (PCTs) have some responsibility for controlling drug budgets, or at least ensuring that drugs are prescribed in a 'cost-effective' manner. For 'cost-effective' we should read 'affordable'.

You can see how the conflicts arise. On the one hand in the UK doctors have the National Service Framework document, which makes it mandatory for patients to have their blood pressure controlled, whereas on the other there are 'guidelines' drawn up by learned societies which recommend that diuretics and beta-blockers be used in patients with uncomplicated hypertension. Thiazides and beta-blockers are cheap (see Chapter Seven), but both can produce impotence along with other side-effects, therefore people are reluctant to take them. Because most people do not want to upset their doctors, they may not even own up to having stopped the medication. This is in nobody's interest.

The cost of treating hypertension is really minimal compared to the cost of not treating it. It is estimated that about 9 per cent of GPs' budgets is spent on anti-hypertensive drugs - this is only half the cost of the whole social care budget of treating people who have had a stroke. On a personal basis, even that amount pales into insignificance compared to the economic and social cost to stroke victims and their families.

The National Institute for Clinical Excellence (NICE) set up by the UK government should theoretically resolve the differences between affordability and effectiveness. Many doctors fear that NICE will do the government's dirty work for them by restricting the use of the more expensive drugs and insisting that doctors use the cheap and cheerful ones instead. This is health rationing. To be fair to NICE, they have sanctioned the liberal use of coronary stents and expensive drugs used during stent implantation, whereas many health service managers were seeking to restrict their use in certain hospitals.

My view is that people should never be fobbed off with old-fashioned medications with high side-effect profiles simply to suit a prescribing budget. If you know there are better drugs available with hardly any side-effects and good 24-hour protection, then you have every right to ask your doctor to prescribe them. This would be patient power at its best!

Enough politics! Assuming you have a good relationship with your GP or consultant and you are prescribed a modern anti-hypertensive, then there is little to choose between them. It is often a case of if 'eye of frog' doesn't work, then let's try 'toe of newt with a dose of wing of bat' thrown in! In other words, it may take time to find a cocktail that agrees with you and that is also effective. It does not really matter if it takes up to six months to bring blood pressure under control, although many people do find it quite frustrating to have their tablets frequently changed. As long as doctors give each drug a reasonable chance to work, and do not make premature decisions to stop one drug and start another, then this patience is well worth it. Doctors must persevere with their treatment plan and not react like the financial markets with actions based on panic and with little or no rational thought.

Side-effects

When you open your packet of anti-hypertensives, you may well be alarmed by the list of potential side-effects which you will find on the piece of paper inside. The list of side-effects may be terrifying, but the manufacturers are legally obliged to put these in even though most of the side-effects will be very rare. In Chapter Seven I discussed the common side-effects that can accompany each drug. Side-effects can be divided into two classes. The first are predictable ones; the second are idiosyncratic. Predictable side-effects will include wheezing and cold extremities (hands and feet) in people given beta-blockers, and a cough in 15-20 per cent of patients on ACE-inhibitors. Your doctor should warn you about these.

Idiosyncratic side-effects are those that are totally unpredictable. In the same way that some patients may have an allergic reaction to lobster or nuts, patients may experience idiosyncratic side-effects because any drug can cause any side-effect in any patient. If a particular drug makes you sprout antlers or turns your hair green, this may be something totally unpredictable, but the antlers will probably drop off once you stop the drug. It is very tempting to blame any symptom on a tablet you are taking, but sometimes this is unfair on the medication. The only way to see if a drug is causing an unusual side-effect is to stop it temporarily and see what happens.

One side-effect I referred to in the last chapter which needs a bit more detail is impotence. Doctors recognise that thiazide diuretics and beta-blockers can cause impotence. There does not appear to be a consistent effect on sexual function with the use of the ACE-inhibitors, the calcium channel-blockers or the angiotensin II receptor-blockers. The alpha-blockers might even improve sexual function. We must remember, however, that impotence has several other causes which cannot always be blamed on the anti-hypertensive drugs. Psychological factors such as anxiety and overwork can cause impotence, as can excess alcohol, diabetes, and abnormalities of the arterial supply and the venous system of the penis. Falling testosterone levels with increasing age can lead to loss of libido and sexual function, and poor sexual function may, of course, be worsened by thiazides or beta-blockers. Some men are naturally shy and reluctant to discuss these problems with their doctors, but these self-inflicted taboos should really be flung aside as there are several ways of helping the problem apart from changing the anti-hypertensive.

Please remember that anti-hypertensive medication is not like a course of antibiotics where 10 days or so of treatment will kill the infection and then the treatment can be stopped. If your doctor gives you a prescription for a month, you must when the month is over go along and renew it. The anti-hypertensives will not work if they sit in their bottles, only if you take them. I continue to be amazed by the number of people who think they only need to take the pills for a week or two and their high blood pressure will be cured.

Monitoring

It is just not good enough for doctors to prescribe an anti-hypertensive drug and send their patient into the big wide world without monitoring the effects of their treatment. Most GPs now have nurses or other health professionals who are trained to take blood pressure, so going back to the surgery to have your blood pressure taken should not mean having to make an appointment three weeks in advance for the GP to do it. However the practice nurse can only check your blood pressure if you actually go along to the surgery - so both you and your general practice surgery have a shared responsibility to monitor your response to any treatment. Of course it may be inconvenient for working people to go to their GP's surgery during the day, but your blood pressure can just as easily be checked by the occupational health nurse at work if there is one.

If you want to check your blood pressure at home, then you may like to consider buying an automatic machine. The OMRON is the most accurate one, having passed validation tests by the British Hypertension Society. Please do not go out and spend a lot of money on an all-singing, all-dancing machine with flashing lights and beeping noises - some of these have not been tested for accuracy.

The 24-hour blood pressure-monitor can, and some would argue should, be used to assess the effects of treatment and to make sure that protection is being supplied for 24 hours or even beyond. The graphs in Chapter Five showed just how vital it is to avoid the early morning surges in pressure. The following three graphs show the 24-hour print-outs for a young woman with severe hypertension, before treatment, six weeks after starting treatment, and six weeks after the dose was increased.

Figure 8.1 shows elevated readings before treatment. The computer print-out told us that 88.8 per cent of her systolic readings and 95.8 per cent of her diastolic readings were abnormal.

Figure 8.2 shows how the patient responded to treatment, but close inspection of the trace shows that the diastolic readings in particular are not yet good enough. The computer print-out showed that now 14.2 per cent of her systolic readings and 38.5 per cent of her diastolic readings were abnormal.

Figure 8.3 shows that after further modification of treatment we are nearly there. Only 4.0 per cent of the patient's systolic readings and 17.5 per cent of her diastolic readings are now abnormal. This patient is being monitored closely to try to achieve perfect control of her blood pressure.

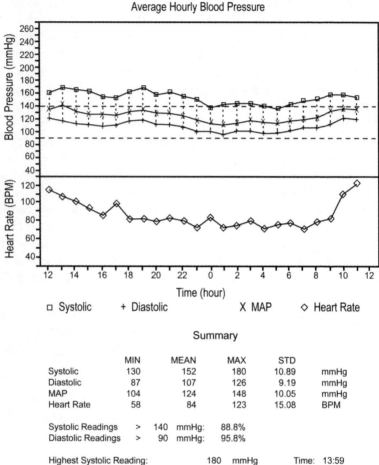

Figure 8.1

24-hour blood pressure monitor print-out showing unacceptably high readings from a young female hypertensive. Before treatment.

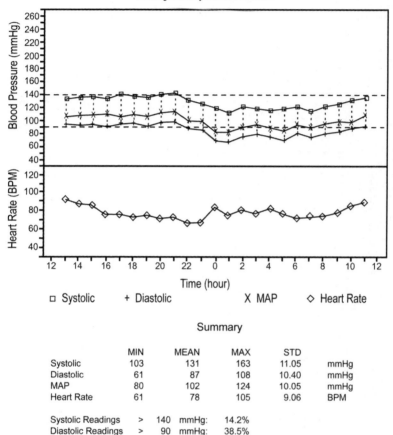

Figure 8.2

Six weeks after treatment.

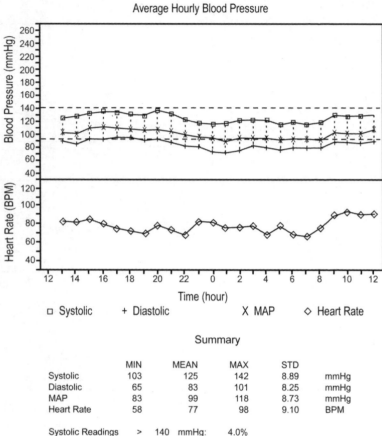

Figure 8.3

Six weeks after further dose adjustment.

Missing a Dose

What should you do if you inadvertently miss a dose? The answer is: first, try not to - but, if you do, please do not take double the dose next time, just take your next tablet at the appropriate moment. Many of the newer medications actually have a duration slightly longer than 24 hours, and some research - particularly with angiotensin II receptor-antagonists - has shown that if a person inadvertently misses out a tablet one morning, he or she still doesn't get the surge in blood pressure that could be so dangerous. This should not be seen as a sign of encouraging you to miss doses. It is just a fail-safe.

How Low Should We Aim to Reduce Blood Pressure?

In 1998 a trial called the Hypertension Optimal Treatment (HOT) Trial was published. In this trial, which tracked 18,790 people, the perfect blood pressure at follow-up was 139/83. In practical terms it would seem that, in people without diabetes, reducing blood pressure to 150/90 would be acceptable as a minimum recommended standard. The optimal blood pressure would be less than 140/85. The British Hypertension Society guidelines from 1999 recommend that for people with diabetes the minimum standard should be less than 140/85, with the optimal at less than 140/80. Why? Because for people with diabetes, lowering the diastolic blood pressure from 90 to 80 will halve the incidence of heart attacks and strokes. People with diabetes, of course, have an extra tendency to develop vascular disease. Being really single-minded in treating high blood pressure aggressively in people with diabetes does seem to be beneficial for them. In order to achieve these levels of blood pressure it is highly likely that combination therapy will be necessary. In the HOT trial, 70 per cent of the patients required more than one drug to achieve the target level.

Combination Therapy
As I have described, most of the first-line drugs are very effective and safe, providing your doctor avoids drugs that are absolutely contraindicated by your condition. I have also described how

combination therapy using smallish doses of more than one drug reduces the likelihood of side-effects compared to giving one drug in massive doses.

There are several possible combination medications your doctor may give you:

An ACE-inhibitor ('-pril') or an angiotensin receptor-blocker ('sartan') can both be combined with a diuretic with good effect. They can also be combined with one of the calcium channel-blockers. Beta-blockers can be given with a water pill or a calcium channel-blocker ('-ipines'). Doctors might not want to give Verapamil and a beta-blocker (Chapter Seven), and neither the ACE-inhibitors nor the angiotensin receptor-blockers tend to work terribly well in combination with a beta-blocker. Another combination doctors try to avoid is one of the '-ipine' drugs and a diuretic.

If a third drug needs to be added, then often one of the alpha-blocking drugs ('-azosins') may be effective.

A Word of Caution
If your doctor changes your medication, please ensure that you take only the drugs that the doctor wants you to take and stop the old ones. In hospital medicine, doctors always like people to bring their pills with them. I have lost count of the number of times I have found people taking two different beta-blockers or two different ACE-inhibitors, or an ACE-inhibitor plus a receptor-blocker and two different calcium channel-blockers. It is a wonder that these people can stand upright at all. Often my only contribution in situations like this is to throw the redundant medications emphatically into the rubbish bin!

Sometimes this problem is caused by poor communication between doctor and patient, so that it is not made clear which medications are to cease and which are to continue. I am also afraid that sometimes patients do not listen. It also does not help if a person goes to two or three different doctors who chop and change the medication without necessarily communicating with each other. In defence of my profession it is not helpful if people go and seek second and third opinions, keeping each of their medical advisers in the dark about the others!

Resistance to Medication

Although the 'eye of frog and toe of newt' principle holds true for most patients, many doctors are now aware that people of African descent respond rather differently to anti-hypertensives than patients of different ethnicities. A particular characteristic of hypertension in Afro-Caribbeans is that it is associated with low plasma renin levels, and hence lower levels of angiotensin II. For this reason the ACE-inhibitors and the angiotensin II receptor-blockers are much less effective for Afro-Caribbeans. Beta-blockers are also less effective, probably for a similar reason. Until fairly recently, doctors just used to go on increasing the dose of drugs for these patients, and often wrongly accused them of not taking their tablets because they failed to respond. We are now more enlightened. Afro-Caribbean people tend to respond better to calcium channel-blockers or alpha-blockers, sometimes in combination.

Despite doctors' best efforts, there are some people who only take their tablets irregularly or do not take them at all. This may just be due to forgetfulness, in which case doctors should ask whether the treatment regime is too complicated for them and perhaps try to simplify it. Sometimes a relative can be recruited to help put out the medications at the right time of the day. Sometimes, however, doctors encounter people who just refuse to take their tablets despite their protestations. In these cases doctors may ask a relative or friend of the patient to look at the bottle or packet of tablets and check they are being taken. Although this may seem to be a sneaky trick, there really are no prizes for challenging fate to give you a heart attack or stroke.

Other causes of resistance to anti-hypertensives include excess salt intake or a secondary cause such as renal artery stenosis or a glandular abnormality.

To end this chapter on a positive note, let me remind you that successful treatment of high blood pressure not only leads to a reduction in strokes, heart attacks and kidney failure, but there is now good evidence that the abnormal thickening of the heart muscle that accompanies hypertension may well reduce. The evidence is particularly convincing for the ACE-inhibitors and the angiotensin II receptor-antagonists. Reduction of thickening of the heart muscle reduces the risk of subsequent heart failure. If I might adapt the old saying, 'A blood pressure pill (or two) a day keeps the stroke unit or the heart failure clinic away.'

Chapter Nine

Hypertension in Pregnancy, the Menopause and in the Elderly

High Blood Pressure in Pregnancy

It is widely known that many women develop high blood pressure during pregnancy. The vast majority of women of childbearing age are otherwise completely healthy, and most will never have had their blood pressures taken before pregnancy. No one really knows what causes some women to develop hypertension in pregnancy. It is a baffling medical condition. The good news is that most women who develop mild elevations of blood pressure during pregnancy will do extremely well in the long term without any drugs, and their blood pressures usually settle back to normal after delivery.

The conditions known as *pre-eclampsia* and *eclampsia*, associated with high blood pressure in pregnancy, are much more serious, though fortunately much less common.

Pre-eclampsia is diagnosed if the mother develops protein in the urine with an elevation of blood pressure above 140/90 in the second half of her pregnancy. Another feature of pre-eclampsia is fluid accumulation in the tissues, known as oedema. However, some swelling of the ankles is common in pregnancy, so this sort of swelling is a less reliable sign of anything amiss.

Eclampsia is a major obstetric and medical emergency, which can have a very poor outcome for both mother and baby. In eclampsia there is marked elevation of the blood pressure, heavy leakage of protein into the urine, and there may be severe swelling of the limbs, fluid on the lungs, kidney failure and even fits. Fortunately, this condition is a lot less common than it used to be, probably because of better medical care and more careful monitoring of mothers during pregnancy.

Pre-eclampsia does tend to run in families, which suggests a strong genetic basis. It also occurs more commonly in young (teenage) mothers and in women over 35. A woman who has had pre-eclampsia in her first pregnancy does have an increased chance of developing it in subsequent pregnancies, although the absolute risk is quite low. Pre-eclampsia is also more common in women of Afro-Caribbean origin than in Caucasians. It is also more common in twin or multiple pregnancies and in overweight women.

Pre-eclampsia is a specific medical and obstetric condition which probably has its origins shortly after the time the baby is conceived. I will not dwell too much on this condition; instead I will concentrate on the much more common type of high blood pressure in pregnancy, which does not have any associated protein in the urine and which generally has a very good outcome.

The definition of hypertension in pregnancy has caused just as much disagreement among doctors as the definition of hypertension in the general population. One group defines it as a single diastolic blood pressure of 110mm/Hg or more, or two readings of 90mm/Hg or more, at least four hours apart, occurring after the 20th week of pregnancy. Other groups have defined it as a rise of more than 15mm/Hg in the diastolic or 30mm/Hg in the systolic pressure compared with readings taken in early pregnancy. Unfortunately, blood pressure measurements before pregnancy may not be available, so it is hard to be certain whether a blood pressure rise in the middle or late part of pregnancy is a real pregnancy-induced phenomenon or a pre-existing condition. Blood pressure may fall slightly in a woman who had mild hypertension before pregnancy, before rising back to pre-pregnancy levels later on, but if there is no record of her blood pressure before pregnancy the doctor is missing a vital piece of information when making a diagnosis.

There has been very little research done on the effect of high blood pressure on mortality rates for mother and baby during pregnancy. We should be grateful that the mortality rates for mothers and babies are now so low that it is hard to detect the very small impact that blood pressure may have on them. We must also remember that child-bearing women are usually young and healthy and at minimal risk of heart attacks and strokes.

What little information there is suggests that very mild elevations of blood pressure during pregnancy do not increase a woman's risk of losing her baby.

Blood pressure should be measured at least once a month during the first two thirds of pregnancy, and weekly in the last one.

Obviously if the blood pressure rises then it should be measured more often and regular checks made on the urine, to make sure that pre-eclampsia is not developing.

If a mother-to-be is found to have a blood pressure of about 140/90 at the first ante-natal visit, in the very early stages of pregnancy, then most probably she is suffering from mild underlying hypertension and *not* pregnancy-induced hypertension. The doctor will take a full history, focusing particularly on any family history of hypertension. If urine testing remains normal and blood pressure does not rise to 150/100 or above, then no medications should be given. If the blood pressure goes up to much higher levels, the doctor must decide whether the expectant mother should be admitted to hospital and prescribed some medication. I will give more information on the sort of drugs doctors can prescribe for use in pregnancy later on in this chapter.

The good news for pregnant women is that, whatever the mechanism of pregnancy-induced hypertension, whether it be abnormal salt metabolism or an abnormality of the placenta, there is absolutely no evidence that a blood pressure below 150/100 adversely affects mother or baby. There is also no evidence that treating this level of blood pressure improves the outcome. Prescribing drugs for blood pressure below 150/100 neither prevents pre-eclampsia nor reduces the chances of a premature delivery.

Elevation of the blood pressure for the first time in the second half of pregnancy can reasonably be labelled as pregnancy-induced hypertension. Again, a small rise in blood pressure in the second half of the pregnancy, with no sign of protein in the urine, carries a good prognosis, but if the blood pressure exceeds 160/110, then admission to hospital and anti-hypertensive medication is required. The grey area is between about 140/90 and 160/110, when hospital admission is not necessary and the expectant mother can be cared for at home. A few years ago women with blood pressures at this level were advised to stay on strict bed-rest, but this has not been shown to be of any value. It may in fact put the woman at risk of developing blood clots (thrombosis) in the leg veins, and clots on the lung (pulmonary embolism). Working mothers should be advised to give up work, however, and it is possible to adopt a tranquil lifestyle during pregnancy without necessarily staying in bed 24 hours a day! The old-fashioned idea of prescribing sedatives and tranquillisers has fortunately passed; there is no role for these unless the woman is particularly agitated. Sensible restriction of salt intake is advisable and although advice 'not to gain too much weight' during pregnancy may be given, this should be taken to mean a *sensible* reduction in calorie intake, which will help the weight gain to be normal and not abnormal.

In some instances it is not possible for a woman to rest properly at home. In these cases, hospital admission may be required.

Drugs for Pregnancy-induced Hypertension

It goes without saying that drugs of any sort should be avoided in the early stages of pregnancy when the developing baby is at its most vulnerable. Doctors are quite rightly extremely hesitant about prescribing any medication to women in the early stages of pregnancy because of the possibility of inducing abnormalities in the foetus.

Given the reluctance to prescribe during early pregnancy, there is little information about the effects of many drugs on the developing baby, but Methyldopa has for many years been the most widely used anti-hypertensive in pregnancy. It does seem to be extremely safe for the mother, and particularly the baby. This drug may produce lethargy, though this symptom would be a small price to pay for the peace of mind of knowing that one's baby is safe.

There is a widespread reluctance to use beta-blockers in early pregnancy because of the effects on the baby, but Labetalol, which is a combined alpha- and beta-blocker, has been widely used without any known adverse effects.

Let me reiterate that using drugs to treat mild hypertension in the early stages of pregnancy has not been shown to be useful in preventing pre-eclampsia or premature delivery.

Thiazide diuretics have long been regarded as not a particularly good idea in pregnancy, as they may reduce the flow of blood into the placenta. Although they are not regarded as being dangerous, doctors still try to avoid them if at all possible. ACE-inhibitors (the '-pril' drugs) are absolutely taboo in pregnancy, as there have been reports of them causing congenital abnormalities and even deaths in the womb.

Hydralazine (see Chapter Eight) can also be used, if necessary, in the early stages of pregnancy.

Clearly, in the later stages of pregnancy when the baby is virtually fully formed, doctors have less cause for concern about developmental abnormalities. If pre-eclampsia develops late in the pregnancy, then hospital admission is required and the baby should be delivered at a time judged to be appropriate by the obstetrician.

One thing that doctors often overlook when prescribing anti-hypertensives to non-pregnant women is the fact that they might *become* pregnant later on in their treatment. If doctors do choose to prescribe an anti-hypertensive drug to a young woman of child-bearing age, then they must remember that they are potentially exposing a foetus to a drug risk. As a rule of thumb, a young woman on anti-hypertensives who might become pregnant should not take an ACE-inhibitor, a calcium channel-blocker or a beta-blocker. The doctor must use his or her judgement before making a decision to prescribe a drug in women of child-bearing age, particularly if the level of hypertension is fairly mild. Where possible, the lifestyle measures I've described - salt restriction, weight loss and exercise, for example - might help keep blood pressures at satisfactory levels without the need to resort to drug therapy until the child-bearing years have passed.

After delivery, hypertension due to pre-eclampsia usually settles to normal within a few days, when medications can be withdrawn. Occasionally, blood pressure remains elevated for some weeks or months, and those women who had undiagnosed essential hypertension before they became pregnant may need to continue medication indefinitely.

The Menopause

Blood pressure will tend to rise with advancing age, so menopausal women may have higher blood pressures than they did in their child-bearing years. As it seems that oestrogens may confer a protective effect on blood vessels, menopausal women who have other risk factors for developing heart attacks and strokes, such as smoking, hypertension, high cholesterol or diabetes, would be at increased risk of heart attacks and strokes after the menopause.

Although it has not been proved that the use of hormone replacement therapy (HRT) reduces the risks of vascular catastrophes back to pre-menopausal levels, there has been enthusiasm for the use of HRT. This enthusiasm has been dampened by the very recent research from the USA that showed an increase in heart attacks and strokes in women taking one particular type of HRT. Many doctors are reluctant to give hypertensive women HRT, but there is really no good reason for this. There is no good evidence that HRT raises blood pressure - although a hypertensive woman on HRT should, like any other hypertensive woman, have her blood pressure checked three or four times a year.

Blood Pressure in the Elderly

For the purposes of medical research, it seems that anyone over the age of 60 is classified as 'elderly', but I firmly believe that this is completely inappropriate in the 21st century. One could argue that even 70-year-olds should not be regarded as elderly. Whatever the definitions, the facts of life are that more and more people are living to well beyond three score years and ten. Blood pressure rises with increasing age (see page 18) - in developed societies if not in primitive rural ones. This means that there are more and more people at risk from the consequences of high blood pressure in later life. If we accept the definition of hypertension as greater than 160/90, then over half the UK population over the age of 65 is hypertensive!

Another myth of medicine which has only recently been discredited is that older patients actually needed higher blood pressure to keep the blood flowing through their stiff and inelastic arteries. This was often used as justification not to treat high blood pressure in the elderly. We now know that this concept is completely wrong. Cynics might argue that myths like these have been perpetuated to discourage giving expensive drugs to older people. We will never entirely abolish discrimination from many aspects of human life; however, by pointing out the facts and the results of several large and well-conducted trials, we can help the medical community understand that the treatment of hypertension in older patients is of great benefit in the prevention of heart attacks and strokes.

A newly diagnosed hypertensive in his or her seventies, eighties or beyond is unlikely to be subjected to the same rigorous investigations in the search for a secondary cause that would be recommended for a younger patient. The vast majority of elderly people with newly diagnosed hypertension will not have rare glandular tumours, but some of them will have renal artery stenosis. It is just not practicable to try to investigate every single patient for this condition, but there are one or two clues. People with renal artery stenosis may well have diabetes, they may have evidence of generalised disease throughout the arterial tree with poor circulation to the legs, they may have evidence of narrowed arteries in the heart or in the brain, and many of them will be smokers.

No patient under the age of 80 should be fobbed off by their doctor with comments such as 'There is no evidence that treating blood pressure is of any use at your age' or similar remarks. There are a large number of clinical trials which have shown comprehensively that treating hypertension in the elderly is beneficial. The European Working Party on hypertension in the elderly looked at 840 patients between the ages of 60 and 99, and compared treatment with a diuretic to no treatment at all. There were 48 heart attacks and 32 strokes in the treated group, and 59 heart attacks and 48 strokes in the non-treated group. These results prove that treatment is beneficial.

A Swedish trial of old people with hypertension published in 1991 also produced positive results. The Medical Research Council Trial of Hypertension in the Elderly (1992) showed a 25 per cent reduction in strokes and a 19 per cent reduction in heart attacks in patients taking anti-hypertensives, compared to those taking dummy tablets (placebos).

There are still a large number of trials, including one called the 'Hypertension in the Very Elderly Trial' (HYVET), trying to decide whether there are benefits in treating hypertension in patients over the age of 80. The trial so far has not been totally conclusive in this age group.

Isolated Systolic Hypertension

One particular form of hypertension that occurs in later life is known as Isolated Systolic Hypertension, or I.S.H. In this condition, the diastolic readings are completely normal but the systolic readings are high. Figure 9.1 shows a 24-hour blood pressure-monitor from a patient with I.S.H, where 84.7 per cent of systolic readings, but only 6.5 per cent of diastolic readings, were abnormal.

Unfortunately, I.S.H. is often ignored by medical practitioners. The two myths that diastolic pressure is more important than systolic, and that older people need higher pressures, are at least partly responsible for this. The statistics show that ignoring this condition is completely wrong, however. Figure 9.2 shows that the risk of heart attacks is higher in the presence of I.S.H. in *any* group, but particularly high in those patients aged between 75 and 84.

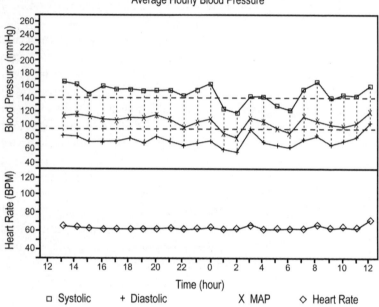

Figure 9.1

24-hour blood pressure monitor print out from a patient with Isolated Systolic Hypertension. Note how during the daytime hours the large majority of the systolic recordings are above 140mm of mercury (squares) but the diastolic readings are all below 90mm/Hg.

The results of treating patients with raised systolic but normal diastolic pressures have helped to eliminate the myth that the diastolic pressure is more important than the systolic. 'The Systolic Hypertension in the Elderly Programme' (SHEP) looked at just under 5,000 people aged 60 or more, who were randomly given either a diuretic or placebo. The treatment was for those people who had a systolic pressure of more than 160mm/Hg and a diastolic below 90mm/Hg. People in the diuretic group had marked reductions in the systolic pressure compared to the people on placebos. After five years of treatment there were huge reductions in the incidence of both heart

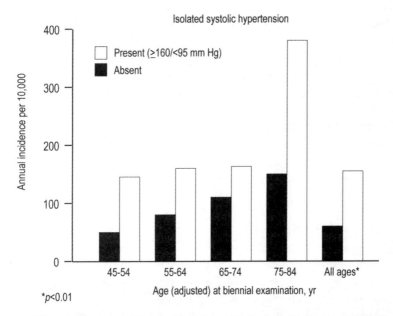

Risk of myocardial infarction with isolated systolic hypertension in the Framingham Heart Study.

Figure 9.2

Graph from the Framingham Study showing how I.S.H. increases the risk of heart attacks in all age groups, but particularly in the elderly. The black columns are those without I.S.H. and the white columns are those suffering from I.S.H.

From American Heart Journal *1999, by permission*

attacks and strokes, and a lower incidence of heart failure, in the people on diuretics.

The results of this trial were confirmed by another trial from Europe published in 1997, which looked at just under 4,700 patients divided into two almost equal groups. One group received anti-hypertensive medication, the other group received a placebo. The study was stopped because of a 42 per cent reduction in strokes and a 30 per cent reduction in heart attacks in the treated group.

The message from these two trials is that no middle-aged or elderly person should be denied treatment just because 'only the top reading is high'!

When it comes to treatment, older people should be given the same advice as the young. A reduction in salt intake, together with weight loss, are advised, although from a practical point of view it is often just not possible for elderly people to get much exercise, because of mobility problems, poor transport facilities and lack of resources. In addition, many elderly people live on their own and eat a poor diet. Surviving on tinned foods is not conducive to the low-salt, high-potassium diet that is good for blood pressure. Those caring for elderly people with hypertension should ensure that they eat plenty of fresh fruits and vegetables.

Drug Treatment

When considering drug treatment in older people, doctors should take into consideration that the patient's kidneys may not be as efficient as they were in early life. Drugs that are excreted by the kidneys may accumulate in the body, and so the doses need to be lower in older people. Also, the reflexes which adjust blood pressure when the body moves from lying down to standing up may be slower in older patients. This can produce dizziness on standing. This is a very common symptom in the elderly and can be made worse by the use of certain medications. Doctors should start with lower doses in elderly people, then the same rules of prescribing apply as with younger patients.

There is evidence that the ACE-inhibitor drugs may be less effective when used on their own in older patients, but are very effective when combined with a diuretic. When ACE-inhibitors or the angiotensin receptor-antagonists are used in elderly people, then blood tests to check on kidney function should be carried out before starting treatment and after two or three weeks, because both these groups of drugs can cause kidney problems in people with renal artery stenosis.

Although we tend to think of erectile dysfunction as a condition which is only distressing to younger men, we must remember that anti-hypertensives can also upset the sex life of older men. Sexual activity is not necessarily less important to a 70-year-old than to a 45-year-old!

Chapter 10

The Truth about Cholesterol and Cholesterol-lowering Drugs

Why am I including a chapter on cholesterol and its treatment in a book about high blood pressure? Many people with high blood pressure are found to have abnormally high cholesterol readings, and if we are to do our best to prevent heart attacks and strokes, then *all* the risk factors must be controlled, not just one of them.

If you turn back to Figure 5.2 on page 42, you will see how important additional risk factors are. Having two risk factors causes a huge increase in the likelihood of a heart attack or stroke. Three risk factors are even worse. The risk is cumulative, so that one plus one equals three, not two! Many hypertensive people will be advised to take a cholesterol-lowering drug in addition to their blood pressure pills; therefore it is worth exploring the reason for this advice.

Serum Cholesterol and Coronary Artery Disease

Doctors have recognised the link between a raised serum cholesterol level and coronary artery disease for a long time. Not surprisingly, a great deal of research time and money has been invested into reducing mortality rates from coronary disease by lowering serum cholesterol. It was logical to start reducing cholesterol using dietary changes. Some of the earliest trials manipulated the diets of people in the study by reducing their fat content, and compared the incidence of heart attacks and death with those of people on a normal 'control' diet. Disappointingly, and despite reductions in blood cholesterol levels, none of these trials showed any convincing benefit of diet in saving lives. Unfortunately the trials were seriously flawed in many ways. They recruited too few people to show an effect, and the diets were often so unpalatable that the subjects did not stick to them and cheated. In addition, many people who had their diets altered changed some other aspects of their lifestyles - such as stopping smoking and taking more regular exercise

- which confounded the results even further!

Later on, trials with medications focused on the effects of lowering cholesterol based on what the arteries looked like on x-ray tests, or angiograms. Researchers had hoped to see the fatty deposits in the arteries shrinking or even disappearing altogether, but this did not happen. Nevertheless, despite the failure of the angiograms to show any discernible changes, there was a tendency for reduced heart attack rates and death rates in the treated groups, but nobody really understood why.

It is only since the discovery of the mechanisms by which arteries fur up and by which heart attacks occur that the role of cholesterol-lowering drugs in preventing heart attacks and deaths has become clearer. Many of us had in our minds an image of arteries passively furring up as cholesterol and other fatty compounds gently deposit on the artery walls, a bit like mud and silt slowly settling on the floor of a slowly flowing stream or canal. It has been tempting to think of cholesterol making the blood thicker and more viscous, so that patients with high cholesterol levels have more 'treacly' blood that silts up quickly. This concept is attractive but, put bluntly - completely wrong! We now know that arteries do not passively silt up, but that atheroma and arterial narrowing occurs as an *active* process, as a result of inflammation and injury to arterial walls. Many people will know that cholesterol consists of two main components - high-density lipoprotein (HDL) and low-density lipoprotein (LDL). In the body, LDL becomes oxidised (oxidisation is a chemical process - when iron becomes oxidised it turns to rust). This oxidised LDL is incredibly harmful to artery walls - it is like poison. It attracts white blood cells, which are part of the body's defence system, and an intense inflammatory reaction occurs. The white cells ingest the chemical and then die, releasing their fatty contents onto the inner surface of the arterial wall. If this process continues for years, the result is a fatty deposit called a *plaque*, which eventually obstructs the artery.

A fibrous cap covers these plaques, separating the fatty substance from the blood flowing through the artery. Many of these plaques remain stable for decades, causing little or no symptoms. A slowly growing plaque in a coronary artery may eventually cause angina when it becomes large enough to reduce the flow of blood into the heart muscle. However, some of these plaques are unstable, and the fibrous cap may be fragile. In an unstable plaque, the fibrous cap may rupture or fissure, just like the ground in an earthquake or the top of an erupting volcano. Suddenly, the blood flowing through the artery is exposed to the fatty core, and when this happens a blood clot may form quickly. Why? The reason is that fatty material causes a chemical reaction in the blood, causing it to clot. Many of these fatty, unstable plaques are too small to be detected by any imaging technique and will not cause a significant obstruction until the clot forms. This explains why so many heart attacks and sudden cardiac deaths occur out of the blue in people who have had no symptoms at all.

Statin Drugs

The newest cholesterol-lowering agents belong to a group of drugs known as the *statins*, which lower both total cholesterol and LDL cholesterol levels by between 30 and 60 per cent in humans. They work by preventing the manufacture of cholesterol in the body, and they achieve this by blocking one of the chemicals, known as an enzyme, necessary for the manufacture of choles-terol. However, this action may not be as important as their effect on LDL cholesterol. The statins prevent LDL being oxidised, and thus reduce the stimulus to inflammation and injury to the artery wall. Put simply, no inflammation means an absence of dying white cells releasing fatty deposits onto the walls of the arteries. It is hard to measure this anti-inflammatory action in a living person, so the only way doctors can test that the drugs are having an effect is to measure the cholesterol and LDL levels in the blood.

These drugs have been subjected to several large, landmark trials for the prevention of coronary deaths. A trial from Scandinavia and another from the US found big reductions in heart attacks and death rates. There was also a reduction in the need for coronary bypass surgery in patients with heart disease and elevated cholesterols treated with a statin, compared to those on placebo (dummy pills). The statin-treated patients also had fewer admissions to hospital. One very important but unexpected finding from these trials was a large reduction in strokes.

By reducing the oxidisation of LDL, the statins stabilise plaques in arteries, and make their rupture and consequent blood-clot formation much less likely. The data suggest that this applies to both coronary and carotid arteries. So, just as blood pressure-lowering drugs protect arteries from the stresses imposed by high pressure, the statins protect them by reducing the inflammation, injury and clot formation.

Trials in healthy people without obvious heart disease have also produced encouraging results. A trial conducted in Glasgow followed just under 6,600 healthy males with high LDL levels for four to nine years. There were fewer heart attacks and deaths in the statin-treated group compared to placebo, although the numbers were very small.

It is universally recognised that statin therapy should be part and parcel of a prevention strategy in virtually anybody with proven coronary disease. Audits of doctors' practices suggest that they are a) not prescribing statins widely enough or b) not ensuring that the recommended target levels of cholesterol and LDL are achieved. A study published in 1996 examined the scope for preventing further problems in heart attack victims, and in those who had undergone bypass surgery or balloon treatment. Information was obtained from 12 cardiac centres and 12 district hospitals in 12 different geographical regions in the UK. Over 75 per cent of these patients still had cholesterol levels of greater than 5.2mmol/l. The use of aspirin, beta-blockers and anti-hypertensive drugs was also too low.

It is clear that the statins are not yet being prescribed as widely as they should be. A major problem in the UK is that many NHS hospital laboratories will not routinely measure LDL or HDL levels in the blood. They produce a level for total cholesterol (TC) and for triglycerides (another type of blood fat). This is exasperating for doctors responsible for deciding who might benefit from the statins. The only possible motive for this failure is to save money. An additional pressure in the UK is that limited prescribing budgets may prevent the use of a statin in the correct dose, or may narrow the choice of drug used. The goalposts for the 'correct' cholesterol and LDL levels in the blood keep moving, and what was regarded as 'normal' five years ago for somebody with heart disease is now felt to be way too high. The medical profession has been urged to work hard to meet the constantly changing targets as more and more research is published.

The largest statin trial ever conducted, the Heart Protection Study, was published in the summer of 2002. This was the first trial to include large numbers of women and patients over the age of 70. The results showed that in anybody who is at high risk of developing heart attacks and strokes, these drugs produce a very substantial reduction in heart attacks, heart related deaths and strokes. So anybody with diabetes, or with any arterial problems anywhere in the body, will benefit from these drugs. The benefits were also seen in patients over the age of 75 years; so let nobody tell you that these drugs have no benefit in elderly people. The study has also made doctors rethink their approach to cholesterol targets, because driving the LDL cholesterol down even lower than the current target levels provided a massive extra benefit in terms of lives saved and in heart attacks and strokes prevented.

People who are prescribed statins should be reassured about the safety of the ones currently on the market. Among the myths and rumours that all drugs have to contend with is the notion that these drugs cause madness and suicide. In the Heart Protection Study, there was no increase in the incidence of malignant tumours or suicide. Information on the safety of statins may be found on-line at www.nhlbi.nih.gov/guidelines/cholesterol.

In Summary

For people with high blood pressure, doctors should forget about targets for cholesterol and LDL, and focus instead on how to reduce the total risk of heart attacks and strokes. If this means that you have to take one more pill each day to keep you well - then so be it. When humanity needs fewer people like me to attend to their heart problems - then we will have done our jobs well!

Conclusions

We know *how* hypertension is caused, but we do not know *why*. We know how to *treat* it, but not how to *cure* it. A cure may require some sort of gene therapy and doubtless will come some day, probably before a cure for the common cold!

In our imperfect, disease-ridden world, having a treatable condition is relatively good news. I hope that you will feel encouraged by the positive message that runs through this book: Treating high blood pressure improves the quantity, and hopefully the quality, of life. You will probably gain more from having your blood pressure checked - and treated, if necessary - than from buying a lottery ticket or scratch card!

Helpful Websites

www.hyp.ac.uk/bhsinfo
  *self-help leaflets and information on lifestyle alterations and
some drugs*

www.nephron.com
  American site for those who have hypertension and kidney disease

www.bhf.org.uk
  British Heart Foundation

www.diabetes.org.uk
  Diabetes Association

www.stroke.org.uk
  *information for stroke victims and their families.
  Helpline 0845 303 3100*

www.mco.edu/whl
  World Hypertension League; features articles for the public

www.americanheart.org
  *American Heart Association with several links to sites with
hypertension information for the public*

www.ash-us.org
  *American Society of Hypertension, with a good information
page and useful statistics*

Further Reading

Beevers and MacGregor. *Hypertension In Practice* (3rd edn; Martin Dunitz, 1999)
  Suitable for medical professionals

Acknowledgements

I am truly grateful to Julie White and Joan Christenson for their expert secretarial help and immense patience. Without them and the understanding of my family, this work would never have emerged from my hectic and disorganised life. I would like to thank everybody who has had to put up with my whingeing about deadlines and impossible work schedules. You will have your reward in heaven - but hopefully not too soon!

Index